THE
UNCHAINED
MIND

Overcome Social Anxiety and Unleash True Self-Confidence

The Complete Guide to helping you free yourself from the Clutches of Social Anxiety and live a life full of high Self-Esteem and Self-Confidence!

DANIO KAVI

CalmKavi.com

Visit the Official Website at: CalmKavi.com

Printed in Australia.

First Printing: 04/2024

CalmKavi Publishing

Hardcover ISBN: 978-1-7635285-0-5
Paperback ISBN: 978-1-7635285-1-2
Audiobook ISBN: 978-1-7635285-2-9

CalmKavi Publishing books may be purchased for educational, business or sales promotional use. Special discounts are available on quantity purchases. For more information, please reach out via email.

Email: danio@calmkavi.com

For orders by U.S. trade bookstores and wholesalers, please contact CalmKavi Publishing at the email address listed above.

DISCLAIMER

THE
UNCHAINED
MIND

Why I Wrote This Book

Simply put, I have faced crippling social anxiety myself and I know how painful it is just to step out past the front door of my own house. Over the years, I have gained knowledge and experience with how to deal with this type of anxiety. One of the things that took me by surprise back then, was how many other people were going through pretty much the same thing I was going through. I wrote this book, so that I could help other social anxiety sufferers like myself and teach them how to deal with the anxiety and improve their self-confidence so that they can carry on with and enjoy life to the fullest. I also wanted to collate everything I've learned in a neat, compact and digestible book that will help not only myself, but other social anxiety sufferers. I wanted to provide an affordable resource for sufferers and give them confidence to tackle the challenges of social life by following a series of easy-to-follow steps.

Why You Should Read This Book

This book will help give you the tools and skills to overcome social anxiety. You will learn ways to cope with social anxiety and take back control of your life so that you can live your life to the fullest.

The techniques in this book leverages the proven and widely known technique called Cognitive Behavioral Therapy (CBT). I will teach you ways to make full use of this technique and incorporate it into your daily life. I will also share some of the "secrets" that have helped me overcome social anxiety.

Practicing is one of the best ways to become better at any skill. The skills you learn in this book can be useful throughout your life. Once you master these skills, you will likely overcome social anxiety and gain confidence to tackle everyday life.

This book has been written in a personable way and I share some of my own experiences fighting social anxiety and some of the scarring issues I had to face. Hopefully, you will be able to relate and find this book more enjoyable knowing my personal story.

This book is designed for anyone suffering from social anxiety and is written in an easy-to-understand casual manner. I truly hope this book helps you in your journey to become confident!

Table of Contents

Chapter 1

Understanding Social Anxiety

First of all, I would like to take this opportunity to say a big and mighty congratulations! I seriously mean it too. The fact that you have this book in your hands (or on your digital device), means that you have decided to do something about your crippling social anxiety. That is admirable. You'd be surprised how many people struggle with social anxiety and put up with it for many years but don't do anything about it. Either they're in denial about it or they have been told by others that "it's just a phase", or "you'll get over it eventually". I was that person back then. In my case, I was in denial. A little about that later. The fact that you have decided to do something about it, means you have started your journey in overcoming social anxiety and gaining confidence. In fact, you have just passed the first step; Acceptance!

Throughout this book, you will learn the skills and techniques required to help you cope with crippling social anxiety. We will be using proven Cognitive Behavioral Therapy (CBT) techniques to help us overcome social anxiety. We will then take it a step further and learn ways to develop self-confidence so that you can start feeling positive about yourself. Along the way, I will share some of my own experiences. Hopefully you will be able to relate to some of the stories I will share and perhaps even feel better about yourself!

I know exactly how painful social anxiety is and how debilitating it can make you feel. Even something as simple as checking the mailbox at the front of the house can seem like a daunting challenge whereas for others it's no big deal. The good news is, as long as you practice the techniques throughout this book, you will get better at facing social situations. I truly hope this book helps you on your path to overcoming social anxiety and gaining true self-confidence.

First of all, I'm not a medical professional or someone who specializes in social therapy of any sort. I'm also no meditation expert (if that's what it's called), or a motivational speaker. Thus, I'm not qualified to give you medical advice. I'm someone who works a 9-5 desk job doing coding for a living. I have suffered from social anxiety for many years and only recently have I found a way to tackle this beast.

One of the main reasons why I wrote this book is to collate everything I've learnt and present it in a way that is easy-to-learn for other social anxiety sufferers like myself.

Another thing you should probably know, is that, this book will NOT cure your social anxiety. I don't think any book can to be honest. The only thing that can help you tackle social anxiety is yourself. You have to be prepared to be brave and persistent for a while. This book will only guide you and provide you with the tools to tackle the beast that is social anxiety. It is then up to you to leverage and make use of those tools to your advantage.

Do You Have Social Anxiety?

Before we go ahead and gain a deeper understanding of social anxiety, it might help to understand if you really have social phobia/social anxiety. Below are some of the symptoms you may feel when you are socially anxious:

- Uncontrollable blushing or burning sensation in the face
- Stiffness in your body posture
- Nervousness and shakiness
- Quivering of the voice
- Mumbling when speaking
- Constantly being told to speak up
- Not knowing what to say in conversations
- Not being able to laugh or laughing too much at jokes
- Not being able to eat/drink in public
- Not being able to buy lunch, instead pack your own
- Smiling uncontrollably or not at all when people speak
- Choking when having to answer questions
- Giving a few word responses instead of an elaborate response
- Lack of eye contact

- Sometimes too much eye contact when they speak to you directly
- Fidgety
- Walk too quickly in public and always with a sense of urgency
- Not being able to relax
- Feeling the need to say something constantly in a group conversation. Disappointed when it doesn't happen
- Rejecting invitations by co-worker/friends to go out to restaurants
- Constantly thinking about how you "stuffed up" after some event
- Constantly thinking about how you "WILL stuff up" before an event
- Rarely approaching people
- Sitting in the back of the room, perhaps closer to the exit door
- Feelings of embarrassment, self-consciousness, awkwardness in front of other people
- Heart beats crazily when you feel like a group of people are looking at you at the opposite side of the platform at your train station
- Keep thinking about how you went, although it is mostly negative
- View others as more superior to you
- Avoidance

Note how I underlined the last point; Avoidance. This is perhaps the biggest thing that keeps social anxiety going.

When we avoid, we become more anxious. I'll discuss this later in the book.

What is Social Anxiety?

A simple Google search for "What is social anxiety" led me to the Social Anxiety Institute website. The website defines social anxiety as "the fear of interaction with other people that brings on self-consciousness, feelings of being negatively judged and evaluated, and, as a result, leads to avoidance". This definition is pretty much spot on and a lot better than how I would have defined it. I simply would have said social anxiety is extreme shyness. But being really shy in the company of other people isn't really much of a problem compared to fearing them.

Social phobia is a form of social anxiety disorder. Someone who has social phobia would exhibit excessive and unreasonable fear of social situations. This feeling of nervousness and self-consciousness essentially comes from the fear of being closely watched, judged and/or criticized.

Most of the time, we think that someone is thinking badly about us. You may keep telling yourself:

- "what will they think?"
- "I'm not as good as him/her though"
- "I don't deserve to go to that party because I'm not rich/good-looking/worthy,etc"

These thoughts, although quite negative, are quite common and nearly everyone has said this to themselves at some point. It only becomes a problem when we constantly keep telling ourselves this. By constantly having these negative thoughts, we start to develop a belief that we are "less" than others and that their judgement about us is always more important than our own.

When you felt really uncomfortable at that last party you went to, you were probably concentrating too much on how you appeared to others. You may not have even bothered to notice the other guests. Who knows, there might have been someone else in that party who was also really uncomfortable.

Social phobia is a lot more common than you think, affecting millions of people including men and women. The Social Anxiety Institute states that it is the third largest mental health care problem.

Don't think you're the only one. Many others have felt exactly the same way you have. It's probably not as common to babies and younger children, but it is possible that the phobia could have started to develop at a younger age.

There are a number of situations where you may feel the anxiety. For me personally, I have felt the most anxious in group meetings (especially with people I've never met before), public speeches, speaking in front of small/large groups, parties, shops (especially those big malls), restaurants, walking alongside a busy road, and sometimes even stepping outside my house to check the mailbox. Surprisingly, I'm fine with going to the movies. I guess it's because I don't have to speak with anyone and don't have to worry if others are judging me since it's almost pitch black in there!

Waiting at the counter to buy tickets can be nerve-wracking, but I guess now, booking tickets online has made it much less of a problem.

My Difficulties

[Trigger warning: This section contains descriptions of bullying and traumatic experiences]

When I was young, around the age of 5, I used to be a naughty and loud kid. I see old videos of me being the center of attention at my birthday party and I seemed pretty fearless in doing whatever I wanted to do without caring what anyone thought.

Fast forward a few years and I started school. During these years, I seemed to have changed a bit. I rarely ever contributed to class discussions and each year my class report always read "Quiet and conscientious student."

It was around middle of high school when I started to experience a lot of bullying. These were my most traumatic years as I dreaded going to school every day.

There was one guy who constantly picked on me and I think to this day, he still has absolutely no remorse about it. I struggle, even to this day, to forgive him. He would constantly elbow the back of my head when I wasn't looking. He would punch me repeatedly till I got sore. He scribbled all over my textbooks and homework. He would constantly verbally abuse me with a lot of profanities.

I still remember the worst case of bullying I experienced during those day. It was during lunch. He brought along his friends and cornered me in a busy corridor near a window. He was frustrated with me because I rarely talked. He made me believe there was something wrong with me because I was quiet.

He forcefully pushed me against the window and wrapped the rope, which was used to open the blinds, around my neck. He then squeezed hard. I remember choking for air and suffocating while all his friends would laugh. Some of the passers-by looked sorry but didn't step in and get involved. I couldn't really fight him due to my small build. Eventually, he released me and I remember feeling so humiliated and embarrassed.

There were literally hundreds of other similar humiliating situations I had to go through not from this one guy, but from others too. Oh, I could share a whole lot more stories but it would take up way too many pages of this book. I just remember fearing going to high school every day. It was like prison for me during those 6 years. I never told my parents about any of the bullying until recently.

I believe it was at this point where I was psychologically damaged and had developed social phobia. I was so withdrawn from dealing with people at this point.

I apologize if I bored you with my life story. I felt I needed to get that off my chest and that felt pretty good actually.

What To Expect?

I will now provide a brief overview of what we will cover in each Chapter, so that you have an overview of what's to come.

In Chapter 2, we will discuss thoughts, feelings and behaviors and how they are linked as well.

In Chapter 3, we discuss the factors that keep social anxiety going.

In Chapter 4, we discuss some ways to cope with social anxiety when we are put in an uncomfortable social situation.

In Chapter 5, we look at ways to reduce the uncomfortable symptoms associated with social anxiety.

In Chapter 6, we will describe a systematic way to breaking down the walls of social phobia by employing techniques of Cognitive Behavioral Therapy (CBT).

In Chapter 7, we will discuss ways to gain self-esteem and self-confidence.

In Chapter 8, we will assess everything we've learned throughout the book and finally conclude the book.

Summary

In this chapter, we learned what social anxiety is as well as the symptoms and causes of social phobia. We also looked at a number of scenarios where our anxiety may rise. I also gave a bit of a background to my own issues with social anxiety. Finally, we provided an overview of what is to come throughout the rest of the book. In the next chapter, we will look at thoughts, behaviors and actions and how they keep social anxiety going.

You've taken the first courageous step by deciding to work on overcoming your social anxiety. Remember, this journey may not be easy, but with dedication and perseverance, you can make progress. I believe in you, and I'm here to support you along the way.

Chapter 2

Thoughts, Behaviors, Feelings

In this chapter, you will learn about thoughts, behaviors and feelings, how they're related and why they keep your social anxiety going.

Fear

Feeling afraid is normal. There has rarely ever been a person (or animal) who has never been afraid. It's not a bad thing to feel afraid. We need to feel afraid for our own well-being. Without the Fight or Flight response, there would be many more preventable deaths each year. Picture yourself face to face with a tiger. You would feel fear. No one is going to calmly approach a tiger and say "Come at me." Realistically, your body will start to experience new sensations. Your heart may pump faster, the hair on your skin may stand on end, and your focus and concentration would be sharp on the tiger. You may either run for your life, hoping the tiger won't catch you (although deep inside you know you're in danger), or you will be so pumped up that you will take on the tiger since you have no other option. Animals exhibit this response too. A stray dog may run away if you chase it, but eventually, it may have no other choice but to turn around and bite your leg. This is called Fight or Flight. We either fight to protect ourselves or flee for our lives. It's good that we have this response as it helps keep us alive in times of real danger.

If the Fight or Flight response occurred in non-dangerous situations, it would be problematic. In other words, if our body reacts the same way as when dangling off a plane to simple scenarios like walking into a public shop, then that is when we need to address it. Even though anxiety can be beneficial, one reason why social anxiety is challenging is that the Fight or Flight response unnecessarily kicks in for harmless social situations. Sitting alone at a party, walking along a busy street, or meeting a stranger for the first time will most likely not cause us any danger, yet our bodies may react as if they do. We need to train our bodies to understand that the Fight or Flight response is not required for these mundane situations. That is exactly what we'll be working on throughout this book.

Situations vs. Thoughts vs. Feelings

The root cause of your social anxiety problems is your thoughts. You aren't thinking correctly about situations. I'll explain myself.

Think of a few situations that you consider scary right now, such as standing in front of hundreds of people to give a speech, meeting strangers at a party, or eating/drinking in a public park. The reason you feel socially anxious is not because of these situations themselves. What you fear are your own thoughts about those situations, not the situation itself. Your thoughts about the situation then drive you to behave differently than you otherwise normally would, and feelings of awkwardness, nervousness, embarrassment, and self-consciousness follow shortly afterward.

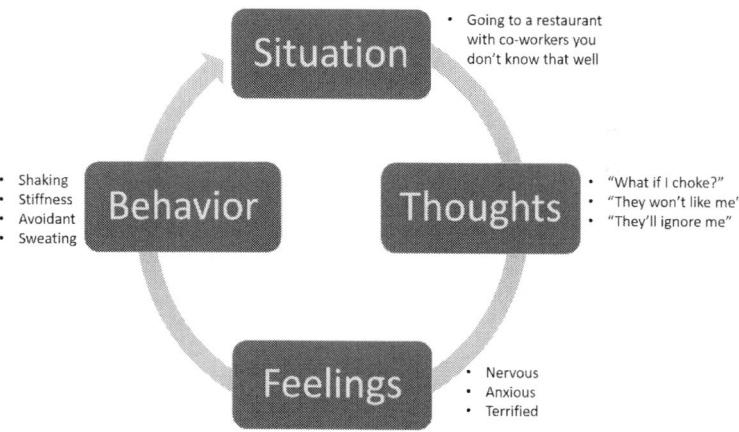

Simply put, the situation drives you to think negatively. Those negative thoughts reinforce negative beliefs about yourself, and in turn, you feel bad. When you feel badly about yourself, you start to act differently.

Let's consider a simple example. Imagine a guy named Tim hears a large bang outside at night. His immediate thoughts are, "What was that? Did someone just get shot outside? Is there a gunman on the loose? I'm going to die tonight. The gunman will target me next." These thoughts cause him to feel worried and anxious. His heart races, and his body tenses up. He then covers himself with a blanket, hoping the gunman won't find him. Now imagine another guy named Bob, who lives next door to Tim. He also hears the large bang. The thoughts running through his mind are, "What was that? Is it the fireworks already? Awesome, I wish I had my camera nearby so I could take pictures. I'm sure it will be spectacular. I'm not going to miss out on this." Bob would then leap out of bed and look out his window to find the source of the sound.

See how the exact same situation created two different reactions from two different people? Tim's thoughts were more along the lines of something bad happening, while Bob's thoughts were largely positive. Thus, Tim felt worried and anxious, and Bob felt excited and eager. The situation itself was the same. The large sound could have been a trash can toppling over due to heavy winds. However, the situation had nothing to do with how Tim and Bob felt. It was simply their way of thinking that caused them to feel differently.

Situation	Thoughts	Feelings
Sound outside	"What was that? Did someone just get shot outside? Are there gunmen on the loose? I'm going to die tonight. The gunmen will target me next."	Worried Anxious Tense
Sound outside	"What was that? Is it the fireworks already? Awesome, I wish I had my camera nearby so I could take pictures. I'm sure it will be spectacular. I'm not going to miss out on this".	Excited Eager

This example can be applied in the same way to a social setting. Let's say Alice, a popular person, has invited both Tim and Bob to her party in two weeks. If Tim has social anxiety and Bob doesn't, their thoughts would differ. Tim might think, "Oh no, I'll look weird and uncomfortable. They're going to laugh at me when they see me standing there awkwardly. I can't approach people. What will they think of me? I don't belong there, I'm not as popular as Alice. I'm not worthy of this. I think I might bail and say I can't come because I forgot my shoes or something." This would result in him constantly fretting about the event, feeling nervous, anxious, and unable to relax until the party is over. Meanwhile, Bob might think, "Oh yeah, I'm gonna love this. I get to meet all of my buddies who I haven't seen in a while. I know I'm going to be hilarious. And better yet, I get to update my Instagram and Google+ since I haven't done it in a while. Seriously, I can't wait!" Since Bob's thoughts are mostly positive, he will be excited to go to the party and will be counting down the days.

Again, the same situation, but differing thoughts have created differing feelings about it.

Situation	Thoughts	Feelings
Invited to party	"Oh no, I'll look weird and uncomfortable. They're going to laugh at me when they see me standing there awkwardly. I can't approach people. What will they think of me? I don't know what to say!"	Worried Anxious Tense
Invited to party	"Oh yeah, I'm gonna love this. I get to meet all of my buddies who I haven't seen in a while. I know I'm gonna be hilarious. And better yet; I get to update my Instagram and Google+ since I haven't done it in a while. Seriously, I can't wait!"	Excited Eager

Could you relate to this? Think of a time you last felt anxious about something socially related. Do you remember what you were thinking during/before/after that time? Could this be the reason why you felt anxious?

If you don't remember, that's fine. This is one thing we will be looking at throughout this book. That's one of the main parts of CBT – really listening to ourselves when we face our fears and analyzing why the way we're thinking is affecting our feelings. We'll attempt to replace negative thoughts with better thoughts. In other words, we'll be washing away all the negative thoughts in our brain and filling it with positive ones. That's how we will tackle social anxiety; with a lot of self-encouragement.

So remember, the way you think affects the way you feel. The situation itself has nothing to do with it.

Negative Thoughts

There are a couple of different types of negative thoughts. Let's briefly go through some of them with examples:

Jumping to Conclusions

This is where you claim something negative happened without evidence. For example:

"I am unlikeable."

"Everyone thinks I'm a weirdo, even people I haven't met. They can just sense it."

Black or White Thinking (All or Nothing)

In this type of thinking, you feel that you have to be completely perfect or you're a complete failure. There is no "middle ground." For example:

"I almost tripped when I walked past a group of people. I completely ruined my reputation and image."

What If

These are the types of statements said when anticipating or picturing something going wrong:

"What if I mess up that speech tomorrow?"

"What if my drink spills while I'm talking to someone at lunch?"
"What will they think of me if I forget to say goodbye at the end of the day?"

Overgeneralizations

If something bad happens once, we expect it will keep happening repeatedly. We start to lose trust in that situation and use that single instance as evidence that it will happen again:

"I choked on one food item at that restaurant; it will definitely happen again when I'm forced to go there next week."

Magnifying and Minimizing

This is where you take a minor bad situation as catastrophically bad and downplay a good situation. For example, you may have laughed awkwardly during a group conversation, causing others to notice momentarily. You might go home and dwell on that the rest of the day and night, wondering why you laughed and how you could have handled it differently. This is magnifying. Likewise, if you get awarded a PhD in Neuroscience and people are amazed at your talent, you might downplay it as if anyone could achieve it with some effort. This is minimizing.

"I was the laughingstock of the whole company today when they mispronounced my last name."

"I came first in this exam, but there weren't many competitive students, and anyone could have come first. I'm really not that smart."

Personalization

This is where you feel that everything others do is directly because of you. For example:

"The manager seemed angry when he walked into his office, did I do something to make him angry?"

"She doesn't seem as cheerful as last week; it was probably my fault since I was quiet, and she thinks I'm cold."

Approval Seeking

This is the excessive need to be approved by others. When others validate you, it is only then you feel validated. You might even change yourself to please others:

"What will they think of me?"

"My day is ruined because a person I just met today hates me. I am unlovable."

Blaming

You blame others for the way you feel, even though only you can control your feelings:

"She was the reason why I couldn't open up; otherwise, I would have been fine."

"He's the reason why I don't make jokes anymore."

Should statements

We make imaginary rules of how we and others should act and feel. When we don't act the way we think we should, we get frustrated, angry, and sometimes guilty:

"I should be more confident and outgoing."

"I shouldn't be this quiet. I should say something to break the awkward silence even though I don't know what to say."

Emotional reasoning

The idea that how you feel must be true. If you're feeling happy, the whole world is happy, and you're the happiest person. If you feel awkward and self-conscious, you believe you are a weirdo that no one likes:

"I feel weird, therefore I am weird."

"I feel like I'm really quiet and uninteresting, therefore I am boring."

Labeling

This is name-calling oneself in a harsh way:

"I'm a loser."

"I'm such an idiot, seriously."

All of these types of negative thinking contribute to your social anxiety. Try to identify the thoughts that enter your mind in social situations and categorize them into one of these types. One statement could fit multiple categories. If you constantly find yourself having these types of negative thoughts, then your way of thinking about yourself and the world isn't healthy, and it needs to change. Don't worry; we will start to change this in the following chapters.

Distorted Beliefs

One reason negative thinking is problematic is that constantly doing this will distort beliefs about ourselves. There is truth to the saying that if you constantly tell yourself "I'm the best at cricket" at least a hundred times a day, you will eventually start to believe that you are the best at cricket, whether true or not. You will have developed that belief.

Try to observe how people talk. Sometimes you might encounter people saying, "I'm probably going to fail. I don't know why I'm doing this. I don't even know what I'm doing right now." Generally, you'd find them quite gloomy and complaining about why life isn't fair to them. When they constantly say this, they start to develop the belief that they're a failure. As a result, they tend to look depressed most of the time. Then there are those who are more like, "I'm going to ace this. I'll be alright. That guy was pretty good, but I think I can challenge him. I might fail, but whatever, I'll give it a good go." You would find they are generally positive and present in the moment. Their body language can tend to be full of life and energy. They've developed a belief that they can back themselves when faced with a challenge.

You'd have noticed that this very much ties into Situations vs. Thoughts vs. Feelings. When you are socially anxious, you might think, "I'm nervous, I don't know what to say, what if I choke? I look weird, I don't deserve to be here." However, your social anxiety issues didn't start overnight. It would have likely taken years. During that time, you would have faced many social situations and had the same negative thoughts about yourself repeatedly. As a result, you developed distorted beliefs that you aren't good enough, that you will mess up, or that people will laugh at you when you pause awkwardly while thinking of an answer. These beliefs are rarely accurate, which is why they are called distorted beliefs. It is these beliefs that make your body language act differently, causing physical symptoms like heart racing, trembling, sweating, etc.

There can be confusion when discussing the difference between thoughts and beliefs. Thoughts are simply what is going through your mind at the moment, while beliefs are the thoughts that you accept as true (even if they may not be accurate).

Why don't we simply change our beliefs then, you may ask? Well, if it were that easy, you would cure your social anxiety within a week. Remember, beliefs are thoughts that we accept as true in our subconscious mind. The accepting part occurs in the subconscious, which isn't as easily accessible as the conscious mind.

Conscious vs. Subconscious Mind

Learning about the conscious and unconscious mind may help clarify the mysteries behind treating your social anxiety.

The conscious mind is the part of the mind where your actions are controlled voluntarily. When you want to pick up a pen, you voluntarily move your hands. When you do math calculations in your head, you are using your conscious mind. Whenever you are aware that you are doing something, it is because you're doing it through your conscious mind.

The subconscious mind is the part of the mind where your actions are controlled involuntarily. For example, breathing, or when you are about to trip and fall, and your hands thrust forward to brace for impact instead of your face. If you have been startled, your body jolts back involuntarily. These actions are controlled subconsciously. It is generally very difficult to control your subconscious voluntarily. With breathing, for example, you could intentionally alter your breathing temporarily, but you are still not in complete control of your subconscious. Your emotions also live in the subconscious mind – your happiness, sadness, anger, and fears. That's why you feel angry, nervous, and sad when you don't want to feel those things. You could allow your conscious mind to take over and consciously smile and tell yourself that you're happy, but if you still feel sad or angry deep down, then the underlying control is from your subconscious.

How does this relate to social anxiety? The conscious mind is where your thoughts live. When you tell yourself, "What if I mess up? They won't like me, I'm not good enough," you are doing it through your conscious mind. The subconscious mind is where your beliefs live. If your subconscious mind accepts the thought that you are "not good enough," then that is what you believe. Your subconscious has learned from your conscious mind and accepted the thought that you are not good enough. Is it true? No way. But that is what you now believe. This belief has become a distorted belief. You've managed to convince your deeper self that you are not good enough. If you now tell yourself, "I am good enough" all of a sudden, it won't work. Why? The subconscious mind has constantly received messages from your conscious mind that you are "not good enough", that it now accepts that thought. Suddenly, when you say you're "good enough", the subconscious mind will pretty much reject it. Most likely, you would have faced a nerve-wracking situation at a party. You would have constantly told yourself that you can't handle the party that you end up believing in. During the party, just to make yourself feel calmer, you then tell yourself rather nervously that you can handle it, but deep down you know you're not doing too well. The subconscious mind is way too powerful my friend. Those who can conquer their subconscious mind can do wonderful things.

That now ties back to what I said earlier. Ok, so you've developed a belief that you're not good enough since you've been constantly telling yourself that. To rectify this, you must reverse this and constantly tell yourself that you are good enough. That's right, constantly. You must say it as if you truly believe it and say it so many times until you've driven your subconscious mind nuts and it can't be bothered to fight it but give you your wish of believing that you are good enough.

The subconscious mind can filter comments made by other people. When someone passes a comment about you, it is done consciously. Say, for example, your belief is that you're not good enough. If someone comes up to you and says, "You are bad at handling turtles," you would likely not feel hurt by that comment. Your subconscious mind holds no beliefs nor cares about turtles - it's just random. But if the same person says, "You aren't good at anything. Go kill yourself," you would now likely feel very hurt. The subconscious mind will not filter out this statement since it matches your belief system and therefore further confirms your belief that you are not good enough.

To overcome our social anxiety, we need to erase all our distorted beliefs in our subconscious mind. It isn't as simple as pressing a delete button. It's going to take time. We will need to use our conscious mind to work with the subconscious mind and change those beliefs. Once you chip away all those distorted thoughts, you will start gaining clarity when in social situations.

Let's move on. The conscious and subconscious mind are very powerful concepts. Throughout this book, we will be using our conscious mind to tap into the restricted subconscious mind, and we will look at rectifying and adjusting some of those distorted beliefs.

The New Model

The revised model now becomes: Situation -> Thoughts -> Beliefs -> Feelings. That is, you're faced with a situation. You have constant negative thoughts about the situation. You then develop distorted beliefs about the situation based on your constant negative thoughts, as your subconscious has learned and accepted them. You then feel the physical symptoms like racing heart, trembling, etc., when in that situation.

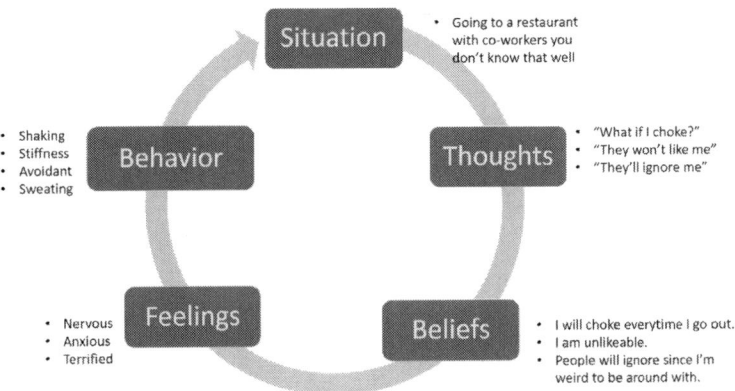

As you can see, this is a vicious cycle that will keep your social anxiety going. You will continue to fear going out to restaurants with your co-workers every time due to this reason. It is only when you break this cycle that you will finally start to drastically reduce the fear of going to these situations. We will be looking to target Beliefs. The way we will do that will firstly be through deliberately and consciously changing our thoughts. We won't be changing the situation, as that is what socially anxious people tend to do through avoidance, which we will explain further in the next chapter.

Summary

In this chapter, we learned about fears as well as gained an understanding of our mind, particularly the Fight or Flight response (which happens mostly through our subconscious mind) and how it shouldn't occur for non-dangerous situations like social occasions. We looked at situations, negative thoughts, and feelings, and how they are related and why we feel uncomfortable during social situations. Finally, we examined the conscious and unconscious mind to better understand why our anxieties aren't easy to fix.

In the next chapter, we will look at what we may currently be doing wrong that causes our social anxiety to persist.

Chapter 3

What Keeps Social Anxiety Going

In this chapter, you will learn the things that will keep social anxiety going. In particular, we will look at fearing anxiety, avoidance and lack of confidence.

Fearing Anxiety

One of the things that can keep social anxiety going is fearing the anxiety itself. Generally, we think it is the situation that we fear, when sometimes, we fear our own symptoms of anxiety.

When you are in a social situation and you think to yourself, "Oh no, what if my mind goes blank, what if I go red, what if I choke, what if I look stiff and weird and so on," you start to fear those symptoms themselves. You fear the symptoms of your mind going blank, your face turning red, your voice quivering and choking, as well as a couple of others. This is generally known as the "fear of fear" or secondary anxiety.

In turn, this prevents your social anxiety from going down, and you start to fear even more. Not only do you fear

29

people not liking you or laughing at you, but you also additionally start to fear how your body will react. There's only so much fear you can take!

For me, it is always group conversations. My voice tends to quiver and sound sort of mumbling and low in volume. I also feel like I can't form proper sentences at times. Like when I need to say something as simple as "I'll eat later," I tend to mess up and make it sound overly complicated and confusing like "I eat a bit like, uh, um...when I have later," which makes absolutely no sense whatsoever. This is one of the main reasons why I stay quiet most of the time. On top of fearing that people might not be interested in what I have to say or think that I'm pretty lame for trying to contribute to the conversation, I tend to also be afraid of myself. It's just a feeling that the next time I attempt to contribute, my voice would definitely shake again and come out weak as usual, as well as my mind going blank.

Avoidance

Avoidance is a bad thing. Like, a really bad thing. Especially for social phobics (if that's even a term). One of the biggest reasons why our social anxiety keeps going is because we keep avoiding social situations. This is never a good thing.

By avoiding social situations, we reinforce the idea that our distorted beliefs are true, in that social situations are dangerous and will always cause social anxiety. As we mentioned in the previous chapter, your subconscious has learned and accepted your constant negative thoughts about social situations. By avoiding social situations, your subconscious never gets the chance to relearn and get that all-important evidence that social situations aren't as bad as you thought they were.

In fact, the more you avoid social situations, the more you fear social situations. When you constantly avoid going to parties, the first time you would believe that you might mess up, the second time you'd think that you would definitely mess up, and thereafter, you would likely perceive parties as a dangerous thing that you should not be a part of.

Generally, the symptoms that you feel aren't harmful at all. It's quite rare that all that heart racing, sweating, and shaking will cause you any harm. As we also learned from the previous chapter, the symptoms of anxiety are a good thing, and we need them when we are in actual danger. Thus, the symptoms are not dangerous, nor are the social situations themselves. People rarely die in social situations. You're more likely to get killed driving a car than being in a social situation. However, when you keep avoiding it, your symptoms become even more uncomfortable, and that is why socially anxious people avoid social situations like the plague.

So, simply speaking, when you avoid social situations, you would very unlikely treat your social anxiety. It becomes part of another vicious circle again. Your fear leads to avoidance, which then leads to more fear, which also leads to even more avoidance. It's a never-ending vicious cycle that just keeps your social anxiety going. It might bring you temporary relief, but it does get harder in the long term.

Your avoidant behavior will only make it harder for you to face social situations the next time.

Avoidance in social situations doesn't have to only mean not turning up to social situations. It can be a lot subtler than that. You could still turn up to social situations and still be avoidant. And yes, this also keeps social anxiety going.

Let's use the example of a party again. Say you turn up to a party, but you are indirectly avoidant. What does this even mean? Some subtle ways you could be indirectly avoidant include:

- Not making direct eye contact with people.
- Not approaching people.
- Sitting somewhere in the corner of the room where no one can see you.
- Taking far too many toilet breaks.
- Staying dead silent the whole time.
- Acting busy on your mobile phone a majority of the time.
- Trying to divert your thoughts about the situation.
- Trying your hardest to remain unnoticed by people at the party.
- It can be even subtler than that:
- Clenching your teeth.
- Smiling/frowning throughout.
- Putting your hands in your pockets because you don't know what else to do with them.
- Facing away from people.
- Looking constantly down.

- Getting your credit card ready before it's your turn to buy a drink.
- Other habits you constantly do to try to feel comfortable.

You might think you nailed going to the party, but you might be disappointed as you don't feel you've nailed your anxiety. These subtle forms of avoidance are known as *safety behaviors*. Safety behaviors keep your social anxiety going.

Completely avoiding social situations as well as subtly avoiding social situations through safety behaviors prevent your social anxiety from reducing. When you avoid it, you might feel relieved temporarily. You have no idea how much it could damage you in the long term. By avoiding it, you will find it harder and harder to face those social situations. And when you find it harder and harder, you will want to avoid it more and more. The anxiety just gets worse. When you avoid all other social situations, your anxiety would seem to worsen for every social situation.

Avoidance was one of the major factors in setting me back from improving socially. I'd avoid all parties, social gatherings, and even sitting in the lunch room with co-workers. When I did get a chance to sit down with them, I would then continue my avoidance through safety behaviors. Things like sitting toward the edge of the table near the exit door, staying quiet and pretending I was interested in what they had to say (when really I was focusing on whether I was "fitting in"), pretending to be busy on my mobile phone, avoiding eye contact, and so on. It gets to a point where you are so quiet all the time that the people in the lunchroom expect you to be quiet. So, when you start talking out of the blue, you seem to leave some of them stunned. Again, that was all in my head. They didn't care if I talked or not. I came to realize after a while that they didn't even really care about me or what I even did. There was no need to put on this fake image in my head of how I should behave. Yet, I continued to be avoidant. Even now, I can be quite avoidant at times, but it is something I'm striving to change as I know that will contribute to the lessening of my social anxiety.

It is important that you stop avoiding social situations. It is only when you stop avoiding that you will start to finally tackle your social anxiety. That's right, you would need to face social situations head-on and drop all safety behaviors. I can guarantee you that you will start to improve, and your anxiety will reduce if you keep facing your social fears and dropping all safety behaviors. It certainly won't happen overnight, but it will eventually happen whenever your subconscious has readjusted and relearned. You will know when your subconscious has changed its mind. It will feel like an "Aha!" moment, and there will be a feeling of relief. Throughout the next few chapters, we will be looking at ways to do this. We won't just tell you to go to a party and just deal with it. That is too extreme. We'll be doing this in a slow and systematic way that won't be too overwhelming. Not to put myself down or anything, but I really think if I could do this, then you could do this better.

Lack of Confidence/Self-Esteem

A lack of confidence and/or self-esteem can also keep your social anxiety going. When you have low confidence, you might find some things really hard to do that other people tend to do without much/any effort. It always surprised me how people could keep a conversation going and how they did it so easily without trying. Back in those days, I remember I even prepared a few questions to ask in case I ever got to be part of a conversation. And here was every other person, just speaking naturally with questions just flowing out smoothly.

Here's something you may or may not know. Confidence comes from being successful at doing something. When you keep being successful at it, your confidence naturally builds up. It just happens. Think about driving. When you learned to drive for the first time, you probably weren't confident driving on one of the main highways. Eventually, you would have had to face the highway even though it made you a little nervous. You would have gained confidence when you finally drove on the highway. As you kept driving on the highway, your confidence naturally grew. In turn, you became comfortable driving on the highway without your parents, with one arm, and with your eyes closed. Actually, that last part would not be possible, and I highly advise you not to try it; it was just a figure of speech. Nevertheless, if you tried to be safe and only drive on the small streets but never expose yourself to the highways, your confidence would not have grown as you would not have had the chance to succeed at driving on the highway. In fact, your confidence may actually decrease if you kept avoiding it and thinking about it later. This leads to the whole avoidance thing.

This also applies to social situations. When you avoid going out to lunch with your co-workers, for example, your confidence will not grow. When you actually go out and realize it's not as bad, you would have succeeded, and your confidence would grow. As you kept going out to lunch regularly with your co-workers, your confidence will naturally grow. In turn, you will become comfortable going out to lunch every week with them without thinking about all the bad things that will happen or whether people are judging you. It will just become second nature to you. You would be able to do it with your eyes closed. Again, a figure of speech.

When you find out you can manage things that you thought were difficult, you build your confidence. Conversely, when you keep thinking that other people will not like you, think you're odd/weird and unlikeable, think you're just plain stupid, and so on, you destroy your self-confidence. You don't need that. When you destroy your self-confidence by thinking this way, you would very much hate any contact with others and pretty much refuse to trust anyone. This creates that vicious cycle we keep talking about:

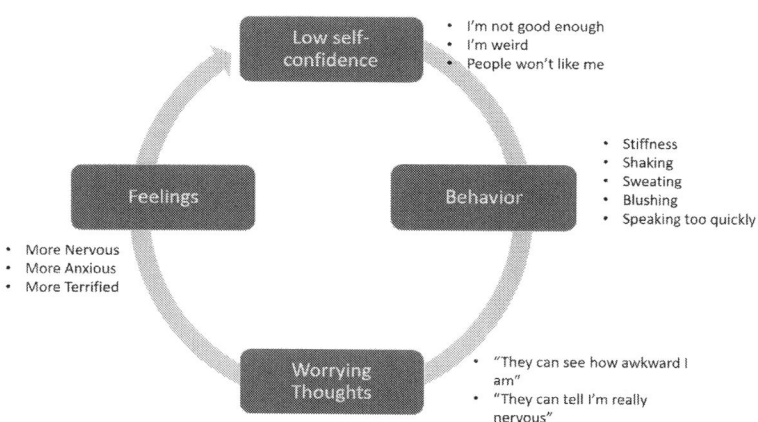

Worrying about how people will react is pretty much what social phobia is all about. This is why when you do things in front of people, such as speaking on a telephone, being interviewed for a job, or contributing to a group conversation, you put yourself out there to be judged. If you have low self-confidence and self-esteem, you would believe others will always judge you poorly and reject you for being who you are. Having low self-confidence and low self-esteem is pretty much like saying that you don't like yourself. When you don't like yourself, you would obviously believe no one else would like you.

It is then pretty obvious that you would likely feel anxious, and then you experience the anxiety symptoms. This then creates the temptation to continue avoidance of social situations as well as avoiding/refusing to show your true self to others. This is very natural, of course. However, as we saw from the vicious cycle, the more you avoid, the more you reduce your self-confidence that you can handle social situations, and so the worry cycle continues with even greater force next time.

Summary

In this chapter, we looked at some of the factors that keep your social anxiety going. We looked at the fear of fear, avoidance, and loss of confidence and self-esteem. We learned that the best way to start tackling social anxiety is to stop avoiding and drop all safety behaviors when we actually decide to turn up. Although it sounds easy to say, it is definitely not so easy to execute. In the next chapter, we will finally start to do something about our social anxiety and look at ways to relax in social situations as well as shift attention away from our negative thoughts.

Chapter 4

Coping With Socially Anxious Symptoms

If you're thinking, "Hurry up and teach me how to get rid of my social anxiety already" and had enough of all that boring theory from the previous chapters, well, we'll finally be doing that. In this chapter, you will learn ways to cope with your anxiety. We will look at relaxation techniques and shifting attention as a first step to reduce anxiety when we are in a social situation.

Relaxation

When you are in a social situation, just relax. You would then find social situations less stressful. Wait a second, "just relax"? That might be the worst advice I've given. The point of this book is for me to teach you how to relax in social situations, not simply say "just relax". It isn't easy for someone with social anxiety to just relax at the click of a finger. Sadly, you may have heard this many times from people who don't have social anxiety. I know this happened to me a lot. I know their intentions were good, but telling me to just relax did absolutely nothing. If I was able to just relax, I wouldn't have had social anxiety in the first place.

Let's get the facts straight. Relaxing in social situations is seriously helpful. It can reduce our social anxiety and make us less focused on ourselves. When we get anxious in social situations, we are not relaxed. We are stressed and very panicky. You can tell from the symptoms you experience, such as a heart racing fast, muscle tension, stiff and rigid body movements, and so on. As we discussed in the previous chapter, these symptoms can cause another vicious cycle where you end up feeling even more anxious and stressed.

When we relax, our anxiety and stress levels become a lot more manageable. When we relax, we find that we are able to handle our social anxiety much better. In essence, by learning to relax in social situations, we learn to control our social anxiety. We show our anxiety about who is the boss!

The problem? Learning to relax is not an easy thing. There aren't many people who can deliberately relax on the spot whenever they want to, even more so when they are anxious. It is possible, however. The people who practice meditation, yoga, and other spiritual-related stuff are able to relax on cue and always seem at peace with the world. We can borrow some of their techniques to help us with our social anxiety.

The Slow Breathing Technique

This is one of the first things you might learn when you see a social phobia psychologist or enroll in a CBT program. The idea with the Slow Breathing technique is to deliberately slow down your breathing rate in social situations so that you drastically reduce some of the physical symptoms of social anxiety.

When you are socially anxious, your breathing rate tends to be pretty fast. This can help reinforce that fight or flight response, triggering the physical sensations.

You might also find that when you speak, your voice tends to be quite rushed, and you may run out of breath, sort of like trying to speak after the end of a running race. When someone would ask me, "How did you find this place?" I would tend to answer, "Uh...um... alright- I mean uh..., I've come here a couple of times, and uh, yeah, so I'm used to it." Towards the end of that, I would sound a little bit choked out as I realized I was losing my voice. The main reason was perhaps due to my very quick breathing rate, which was exhausting me unnecessarily.

When we deliberately slow down our breathing, our physical symptoms of social anxiety are almost immediately decreased. Not only do we not feel as anxious at the time, but we also do not appear socially anxious in front of other people. That vicious cycle would then start to be torn down. You will find that you will be able to get your words in, and that you are less likely to have a panic attack.

Here is the Slow Breathing technique that you can try to follow along:

1. Breathe in slowly and deeply from the nose for 4 seconds. Make sure it goes as deep as your belly.
2. Hold your breath for 2 seconds.
3. Breathe out slowly for 4 seconds.

4. Hold your breath again for 2 seconds.

The numbers here are just a guide. It's not like you have to follow the 4-2-4-2 seconds rule religiously, or else you'll never get cured of social anxiety again. The idea is that you consciously and deliberately force yourself to breathe slowly. Your subconscious may trigger you to breathe quickly, and it's your job to consciously slow it back down and take control. If you're comfortable doing something like 3-1-3-1 seconds, then do that instead. Generally, 6-8 breathing cycles per minute are considered normal and relaxed. If you're getting over 8 breathing cycles per minute, you're probably breathing too fast. The normal breathing rate is 12 -- 18 per minute. Over 20 breathing cycles per minute, and you're pretty much hyperventilating.

I recommend that you first start off doing this privately. You can do this at home in your bedroom or wherever you feel most relaxed. It is better that you master this at home before you try this in a socially anxious situation. It is also important that you practice this regularly, at least 2 times a day for 10 minutes. Keep doing this until it becomes second nature to you. Once you've developed this habit, you can then try this in a socially anxious situation.

Practice! Practice! Practice! You won't be able to relax overnight if you just practiced it in one day. It needs to become a habit that is ingrained in you. It really depends on the person, but I'd give it around about a month before you should start seeing results. You will then start to feel a sense of relief when you are in a social situation. You will also start to feel that you have some sort of control over your anxiety. This is a very good thing.

So that is your homework for this week. Try this out for a week before you move onto the following sections of this chapter and assess how you go. If by chance, this is working out pretty well, try to spend a few more weeks and even try this out in a social situation you consider frightening. It shouldn't be hard. I'm not saying go up to a person and start a conversation. I'm saying do what you usually do, except now you deliberately slow down your breathing when you feel uncomfortable.

Let Go!

This is another technique to feel relaxed and thus cope with your social anxiety. The idea with this is that you literally "let go" of all your anxiety when you notice it is there. Let's take a look at what this involves:

1. Notice your level of tension in your body and ask yourself whether you feel tension or whether you're relaxed.
2. Drop all tension from your body and tell yourself to relax. In other words, wherever you feel there is tension in your body, just drop it completely. You should be like a ragdoll or a lifeless body.
3. Do this very frequently throughout the day. Try to do it randomly and not only when you are feeling anxious.

43

Some ways you can drop tension from your body include:

- Dropping your hands and shoulders and letting them slump.
- Dropping your head back onto the headrest part of the chair.
- Giving your legs space.
- Sighing.
- Breathing slowly (as just discussed).
- Whispering slowly to yourself the word "Relax".

Another similar exercise that I found to be quite popular is when you deliberately tense your body for a few seconds and then just let go and relax your body (on say the count of 3). For example, you could clench your fists as hard as they can and then suddenly loosen them when you count to 3.

Similar to the Slow Breathing technique, you also have to regularly practice, practice, practice! The more you practice, the more likely you will feel relaxed sooner. Again, first try this at home before you move onto social situations.

Do not expect to feel relaxed if you do not practice regularly. You might fail a few times if you try these techniques, but the good news is, you will eventually be very likely to start feeling relaxed and breaking that vicious circle.

As your homework, I suggest you start learning to do this. That is, first start out deliberately clenching your fist and then "letting go" by releasing the fist. Try to do this for a week. Then, try to do this with your whole body. Tense up your entire body and hold it like that. Then, let go and collapse onto your chair like a lifeless ragdoll. When you keep doing this a number of times throughout the day, this will help make you feel calm and relaxed in social situations. You should then go on and try this out in socially anxious situations.

The main goal with the Slow Breathing technique and the Let Go technique is that you learn what it feels like to be completely relaxed and find where the tension in your body is, so that removing it could be easier.

Other Ways To Feel Relaxed

You generally shouldn't keep thinking about your social anxiety and even social life all the time. You need to have time for yourself. You're your best friend for life, really, if you think about it. You are always there for you through the thick and thin of times. You should respect yourself and pamper yourself as much as you can. Thinking about social anxiety and/or ways to cure your social anxiety can be quite draining and de-motivating. At times, we want to get away from all that and live life.

Some ways you can do this and thus help feel more relaxed include:

- Thinking about things in your life that make you feel relaxed. Examples include walking along the beach, sitting and staring at the sunset in the local park, listening to music, visiting family, or feeling excited for the new trailer for your favorite actor's new movie.

- Relax your posture in social situations. In other words, try to purposely sit relaxed and without care. Being tense doesn't usually look good as we appear to be rooted to the ground like a statue.
- Take a nice hot bath at the end of each day.
- Watching films.
- Driving around town.
- Gardening.
- Playing a sport/Exercising.
- And so on, but make sure you feel relaxed.

For me, sitting in a local park amongst fresh air and nature helps to reduce my anxiety and make me feel less stressed. I also enjoy watching a movie at the end of the week, and it also gives me something to look out for each week! I also enjoy watching YouTube videos as well as listening to music. If you do the things that relax you, you will tend to feel calmer and not worry about your anxiety as much. Doing the things you love could also lead to greater confidence.

Shift Attention Away

When you are in a social situation which you deem to be uncomfortable, you tend to think about your physical symptoms or what others may think of you. When you focus on how others might react to you, you tend to become self-conscious, and you fear the worst of their reactions. If their reactions are as worse as you feared, this can ruin your day. When you constantly look out for others' reactions to you, you would feel uncertain and unconfident about being yourself, and you would struggle to handle the situation in a defined manner. If you remember from what we've learned, constantly thinking about others' reactions forms a vicious cycle that keeps our social anxiety going.

How about we start to try and break that cycle and distract ourselves from other thoughts? It makes sense in theory, right? Instead of constantly thinking negative thoughts (like "What if I mess up?", "What if they think I'm weird"), we stuff it up by thinking about random stuff (like "Oh, that chair is blue, never saw a blue chair before", or "Am I the shortest one here?"). By thinking like this, your subconscious doesn't even know what to gather from your thoughts, and can't make you feel anxious. Instead, your anxiety should decrease.

You might think that's easier said than done. True, I guess. You might consciously try to think random stuff, but in the back of your mind, you keep hearing that voice say, "What if...what if...what if...". Just like with the Slow Breathing or Let Go techniques, it just requires practice. Once you've practiced shifting your attention away a lot, you will find it much easier to cope with your anxiety. Think of a little boy who is quite cheeky. I can imagine his mom yelling and screaming at him not to, I don't know, press a button or something. His mind could be elsewhere, and the next second, he's trying to press that button again. Whereas an overly sensitive person might fear pressing the button because of that screaming reaction. One of the reasons for this is that the little boy, perhaps due to his age, has a short attention span and was thinking of other things, so he rarely felt scared to do it again. The sensitive person may

47

constantly keep thinking about the button and thus fear it. While I'm not condoning a short attention span as a good thing, I just wanted to demonstrate how distracted thoughts can change the way we feel.

Let's look at some ways to distract yourself in social situations without appearing rude:

- Pay attention to what's happening in the situation. You could count how many chairs are in the room, find out how old everyone is, see how tall you are in comparison to everyone else, count how many boys and girls are in the room, and so on. This forces you to focus on the external world rather than what you're going through internally.
- Be busy with something. When you find something to be busy about, you will focus on the task rather than yourself.
- Ask questions. When you ask questions, you divert the attention away from you to the person speaking. Don't keep grilling them with questions, however, since they don't want to feel like they are being interrogated by the police.

Of course, there is a fine line between distraction and safety behaviors. If you try to keep yourself busy by playing with your phone, although you are distracting your thoughts, you are still using a safe behavior, which keeps the anxiety going.

Try to use distraction when you are worried and in a social situation. Don't keep distracting your thoughts, or that can generally come off as avoidant and rude.

Summary

In this chapter, we looked at ways to cope with social anxiety. We looked at relaxation techniques. The two techniques we looked at were the Slow Breathing technique, where we deliberately slow down our breathing to reduce physical symptoms, and the Let Go technique, where we stiffen and tense up your body and then suddenly let go. We also looked at shifting attention away from our anxious thoughts in order to break the vicious cycle called Social Anxiety. In the next chapter, we will finally detail a systematic process for overcoming social anxiety.

Chapter 5

How To Really Reduce Social Anxiety

In this chapter, you will learn the truth about drastically reducing your social anxiety. We will first stress the importance of practicing, being persistent, and the benefits of exposing yourself to the situations that you fear.

The Importance of Practicing

The ONLY way you will get better at reducing your social anxiety, is if you put in the time to actually carry out the steps shown throughout this book. You will need to expose yourself to the public. Not that kind of exposure. I mean, speaking with people, learning to say "yes", instead "not this time, sorry", approaching people and those kinds of things. It is completely fine to fail! I believe I may have heard a saying somewhere that, the more you fail, the more you are likely to succeed. When you fail, you build resilience. You become stronger, and you also build knowledge. You now know not to do whatever it is that caused you to fail. You'd be surprised to know how many people are out there who could improve their social anxiety to a very manageable level themselves, but instead resort to things like drugs and medication. Unless they've experienced extreme social anxiety, I find it a little bit sad. The main reason is that they give up after a few failures. They think that they aren't improving at all, when really, they are getting better, even if just slightly. The more you fail, the more you LEARN not to do whatever caused that failure. Thus, the more you build resilience. You may then try experimenting again. And if that fails as well, then try again. Improving your social anxiety really does come through a lot of practice. It comes through failing, persevering and then experimenting again. You can keep experimenting, failing, researching why you failed, and keep this cycle going on and on. It may seem like a never-ending loop but eventually you will reach a tipping point where everything starts to fall into place. Once you reach your first goals, you will feel a great sense of satisfaction. But don't stop there. Keep going with it and make something else. Don't be a one-hit wonder. Aim to be legendary. Knowing and mastering how to speak confidently is great, but knowing how to speak confidently and also approaching people is even better.

When you start out practicing these techniques, you may find it a bit overwhelming. In fact, that's a bit of an under-statement. You most likely WILL find it overwhelming. When you start to expose yourself to social situations, you may be a little daunted at first and your anxiety will go into overdrive. So overwhelmed that you think that this is it for you, death comes shortly after. When I first started to expose myself to social situations, I seriously felt like I was about to jump out of a plane. I was invited to go out to lunch with fellow co-workers and I said "yes" this time. How did it turn out after the experience? I felt it was really bad. No-one spoke to me. I was extremely quiet the whole time. I'm sure a couple of them might have been wondering why I didn't say a single word to them. The stiffness I felt surely made me look uncomfortable and I almost knocked my drink over (That would have definitely made the experience a nightmare). I kept thinking about it for weeks and felt sure I didn't want to do it again. They kept inviting me and I kept going afterwards. I then came to realize that this isn't so bad. I mean, I came out alive and there weren't any bruises on my body. I came to realize that it really all was in my head. I then slowly applied the techniques that I'd learnt regarding coping with social anxiety, and kept at it. I kept failing. I kept wondering why the heck I'm not improving. In fact, I was so convinced that I'm not improving even 1%. But I stuck with it and kept practicing. Eventually, I reached that point where I started to get better. And from that point on, I could feel gradual improvement. Similar to driving a car. When you drive, the car initially starts slow and eventually accelerates faster and faster. Except in this case, it was more like a ship. It started really slow for a while, and it feels like it isn't moving at all. And then, you start noticing acceleration, or in my case, progress.

Think of social anxiety as a skill just like any other. It takes time to grasp the concepts and learn the techniques of coping with social anxiety. Just like playing the piano. You would first start from the bare basics of knowing what note each key in the piano does. Or even more basic than that, knowing the musical scale and notations in general. From there, you keep learning and practicing. Eventually, you will have built up enough skill and timing to finally start creating your own compositions. Coping with social anxiety and gaining confidence is similar. Although, I'd like to think that it isn't as tough a skill as a piano. But then again, I wouldn't be able to play the piano to save my life.

I read somewhere that claimed research has shown that to be able to master any skill from scratch, you need to put in at least 10,000 hours of work. That's 10,000 hours of learning and practicing. In other words, from the point of knowing absolutely nothing about that skill to being able to call yourself an expert at it, will take an average of about 10,000 hours. In that 10,000 hours, you will need to learn, experiment, practice, fail and do this again and again. The more exposure you get to social situations, the more likely you will naturally become skilled at it and won't rely on some book. You may even write your own book about it one day.

10,000 hours is about 417 days or just over 1 year. Let's look at a scenario. Let's say you fear going to a public shopping mall. If you spent all day at that shopping mall, you may feel an overwhelming and uncontrollable sense of anxiety. But say, you forced yourself to stay there all day for a bit over a year and practiced all your coping techniques during that time constantly. Eventually, you would be really comfortable at a shopping mall. The 10,000 hour thing is perhaps more for an actual skill like playing the piano or mastering a programming language or making a movie or something like that. Social anxiety coping skills aren't super challenging and I believe you can get better in less time than that.

I can't stress enough the importance of practice in achieving your goal. Without practice, this book will be of no use to you. While you can read everything in the book and understand it, you won't truly understand it without practicing and practicing since the human brain retains information in the long-term memory when you actually practice and learn for yourself. Reading about it will only retain information in short-term memory and you would likely forget in about a month's time without constantly refreshing. In fact, there are no books in the world that can help you become better at any skill, just from reading the book alone. I can't say I'm an expert at playing the piano just because I read a book about it. I would only get better once I practice it and try out the techniques for myself. This is why I wrote the disclaimer at the beginning. I didn't want to raise any false hopes in thinking you would get rid of social anxiety after reading this book. So keep practicing even well after you're done with this book to become better at coping with social anxiety.

Feedback

One of the things that can help you in your quest for social confidence is motivation. If you don't have enough motivation, you will stagnate and eventually fall back to your avoidant ways. It's always important to stay motivated, especially throughout your learning period. And one of the best ways to stay motivated is to give yourself small tasks and set yourself deadlines to complete (say a week). Feel good and reward yourself in any way once you've completed it. Then go back and do it again. The idea of setting yourself tight deadlines forces you to work on progressing without stagnating. You can always come back to where you were stuck later on. Also, rewarding yourself by taking yourself out to coffee or watching a movie or even spending quality evening time with your loved ones are great ways to keep your motivation going strong.

Another form of motivation and one that can aid in the confidence-gaining process, is feedback. Try to get your friends, family, therapists or whoever you're comfortable with, to give you **feedback**. When you get feedback or comments from another person about you, your subconscious tends to believe them more than yourself sometimes. That's why we get angry and upset when other people put us down. Those who are able to control their subconscious mind tend to believe their own thoughts more than others while someone who is socially anxious, tends to believe others more. This is perhaps one of the reasons why we can be extra sensitive to others' comments about ourselves and also why we may act awkward and uncomfortable around them.

To get motivated to work on coping with your social anxiety, it is important that you surround yourself with positive and honest people. Positive people can help you change your views of the world and of yourself to a more positive one. Their words of encouragement can help question your subconscious and make you feel good about yourself. When you have someone who keeps telling you

"You can do it, you have the makings to be successful in the future, don't let anyone tell you that you aren't awesome" and so on, that person will directly challenge your negative thinking and hopefully convert you to become a more positive thinker. You may even start to come out of your shell around that person. Popular celebrities, for example, get positive comments all the time from everyone. They may or may not be the most talented in that field, but getting positive attention from people they work with, fans, the media, etc. wherever they go makes them super-confident since their subconscious is fed with tons of positive messages. Likewise, when they turn against the celebrity, that celebrity tends to crumble and resort to getting drunk as a way to get back that "happiness". I've seen it happen many times.

In addition to positive people, I also mentioned honest people. Getting positive feedback can be great, but getting them constantly, can make you question the authenticity of the feedback and your subconscious may even start rejecting them. Someone who keeps saying "You're awesome, you're a star" is great when you are doing well. But when you aren't doing well (and in fact, the opposite), it can get annoying and come across as fake. For example, if you approach someone for a conversation the first time, getting feedback like, "That's great, you're doing really well, I'm proud of you. Keep it up!" from your loved ones will be great and help you increase your confidence. But then, when you start getting avoidant and going back to your shell and not approaching people when you want to, getting feedback like, "That's great, you're doing really well, I'm proud of you. Keep it up!" from your loved ones will just sound silly. Deep down, you know you aren't progressing and that feedback would come across as fake.

You need them to be honest with you and tell you straight up that you aren't progressing. You need someone to tell you that you are getting worse. You may get really hurt and upset and perhaps even react but you need to learn to accept it and keep at it. Try to understand why they said that and concentrate and how you could fix it, rather than getting hurt over their comments. If they care about you, they will only say things to help you.

I tend to take comments from others this way too. When people says harsh things about you, it can be hurtful. Try to remain calm and understand why they would have told you that. Most times, you will know whether they're constructive and trying to help you or whether they're just downright bashing (and perhaps slightly jealous of you). Life is unpredictable. You may even get people who are rude and scream at you when you're walking down the street. I guess all that agro stuff is best suited for football or boxing or something, I don't know. To me personally, it shows a great strength of character when I see a person rarely react to someone's hate comment. They just take the points for improvement and move on. Initially, I myself was a victim of a lot of these so-called "haters". I remember being quite upset initially. They really know how to push your buttons and ruin your day. But I guess the more you receive them, the easier it becomes to brush it off and say "heard that one before". It's like they have a dictionary of hateful sentences and re-use those again and again. Take criticism with a grain of salt. Take the points for improvement and move on. Likewise with positive comments, don't feel too overjoyed by them. Again, take the improvements and move on. It's never good to feel too upset or too overjoyed by comments.

The Truth About Your Coping Ability

It's time I told you some truths about coping with social anxiety.

The Truth About Your Improvement

The way we will approach our attack against social anxiety is by using the methods taught in Cognitive Behavioral Therapy (CBT). This is something that psychologists usually make use of to treat people with social phobia. The idea is similar to what we've been discussing throughout this book so far. CBT aims to change the way you think about yourself in an effort to change the way your feel and make you more confident socially. That is, it aims to change your negative thinking into a positive one. As I mentioned before, we will be using the techniques of CBT to tackle social anxiety head on.

When you constantly apply this technique, there is a good chance that you will get better at facing social situations. Your anxiety levels should reduce overall. When I checked Google, there are generally mixed opinions regarding the effectiveness of CBT, but is generally more on the positive side. Personally, I am a firm believer that CBT works. However, many people tend to have misconceptions about this form of treatment. I feel that people who are against it and say that it hasn't worked for them, haven't practiced consistently. I wrote a long rant in the previous section about the importance of practice. If you keep practicing CBT, I don't see how you won't improve. The bottom line is, the only way to improve your social anxiety is exposing yourself out there and learning for yourself that you can cope. CBT does that, but you need to be consistent and you need to keep practicing! CBT, perhaps, tends not to work for those who have serious social phobia issues (such as Avoidant Personality Disorder). As I mentioned in the disclaimer, if you have these issues, you may need to see a good, trained psychiatrist rather than this book. They may give you a better plan tailor-made for you and perhaps also medication.

Let's look at one big reason why people tend not to believe in techniques for coping with social anxiety. Many people think, that by consistently applying the techniques of CBT, their improvement will be like this over time:

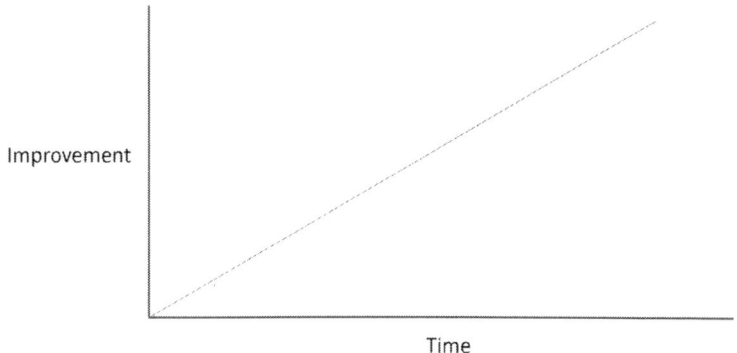

Here is the truth. Your improvement will be more like this:

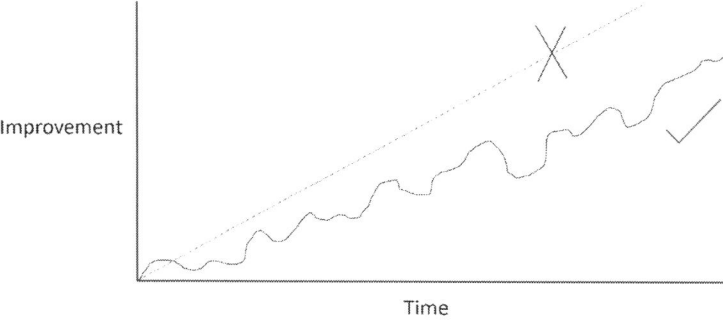

There will always be ups and downs. When you are down, it's important to stay motivated and persist with the techniques. You may think you are getting worse, but you really aren't. Getting worse is a natural part of treating your social anxiety. The idea is that, eventually, your improvement will increase over time. There will be hurdles, but you should gradually get better over time. Sadly, a lot of people write off their improvement as a failure once they hit that first (or second) hurdle. Don't be that person. Just keep at it. Trust me, you will eventually hit that plateau and feel improvement.

The Truth About Your Anxiety

Many times when we are faced in a social situation, we think that the longer we stay in that situation which makes us nervous, the more our anxiety will grow.

There may come a point where we cannot handle this growing anxiety anymore and we leave. For example, when you turn up to a party. You may notice your anxiety levels growing initially. You may feel the anxiety symptoms such as heart racing, stiffness, blushing, sweating and an array of different "What-ifs", "What do I..." thoughts. The longer you stay at that party, you start to notice that your anxiety symptoms get worse and worse. Then, there may come a point where your anxiety level is really high that you can't take it anymore. You'd think that if you stayed longer, you'd either make a serious fool of yourself or that you would harm yourself in some way. It may even feel like you're dangling off the edge of a helicopter and you don't want that feeling any longer. So, you run. You leave the party early giving some excuse. You avoid it. Shortly after, you notice your anxiety level go down almost immediately and you feel relief. The graph below shows you the anxiety level over time that you may experience in these types of situations.

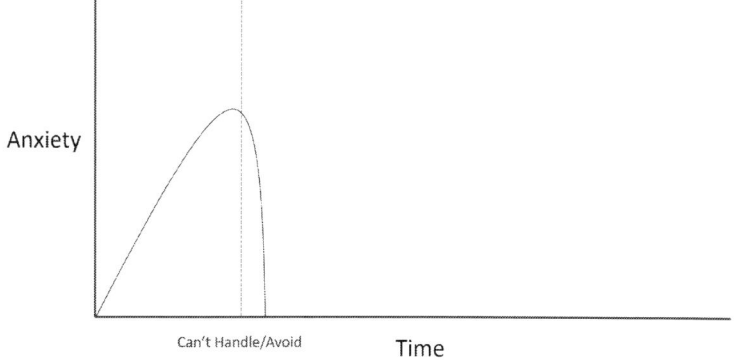

Now, you might think that you have "saved" yourself from harm by leaving early and the immediate relief makes you feel that you survived that helicopter fall without a single scratch on your body. However, you never really learn and teach your subconscious that the party/group meeting/public mall/stranger meeting/etc. is not a harmful experience. Your subconscious will believe that the social situation that you were in is very dangerous. You may think that you were brave for facing the social situation and that you should improve now, but you have inadvertently taught your subconscious to fear that situation more. In fact, the next time you face that social situation again, your anxiety levels would look more like this:

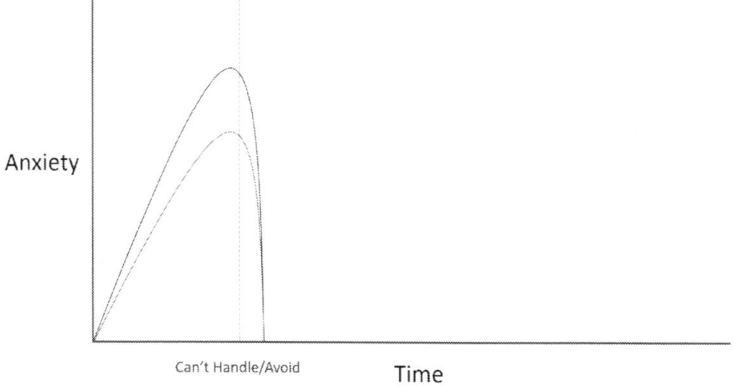

Anxiety

Can't Handle/Avoid   Time

Your anxiety levels would be much higher than it was before. You might have even decided to leave even earlier, which would have done no favors to your subconscious.

See how this influences yet another vicious cycle. Your anxiety levels increase, you don't think you can handle it anymore, you avoid it. The next time, your anxiety levels increase more than before and the vicious cycle continues (perhaps to a point where you completely avoid the situation altogether).

Let me share with you a truth about social anxiety in social situations. The anxiety you feel in social situations are not harmful. Let me repeat that again in case you skimmed that part. **The anxiety you feel in social situations are NOT**

harmful. You won't die or get some unknown mental disorder because of it. Anxiety, in itself, isn't a bad thing. As discussed, it's a part of the Fight or Flight response and it's good for situations when we are in real danger as it keeps us on our toes. We need anxiety in our lives. Thus, what I'm trying to get at is, there is no point in trying to just sit out and "feel" the anxiety in situations that you consciously know aren't dangerous.

Another truth about anxiety is, it reaches its peak and then dies out. That's right! Your anxiety levels may get worse initially. But when it hits that point where your body can't produce more anxiety, your anxiety levels will only decrease from there. It is not possible for our body to produce more anxiety than it can't handle. Our body will produce a maximum anxiety level and after that, it will taper off and fade over time. This is realistically what our anxiety will look like over time:

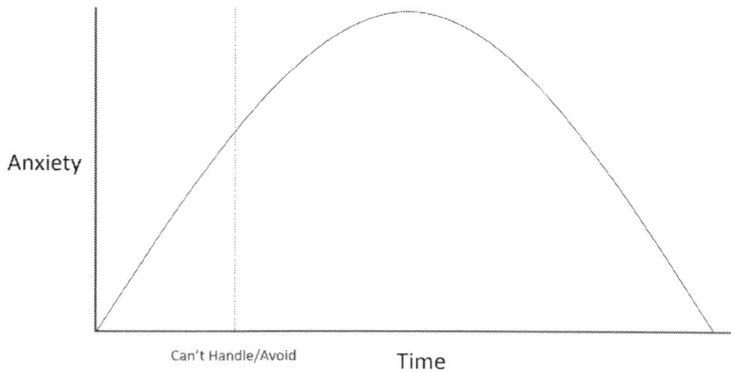

Anxiety

Can't Handle/Avoid   Time

That is, the longer you stay in a social situation that makes you uncomfortable, your anxiety levels will increase to a tipping point, and then start dying out. Eventually, if you stay really long, you will find that situation to be quite manageable. Unfortunately, most people with social phobia aren't aware of this fact. They think their anxiety levels are unbearable to the point that they need to leave before it gets really bad and something bad will happen to their health. They tend to visualize their anxiety being more like this:

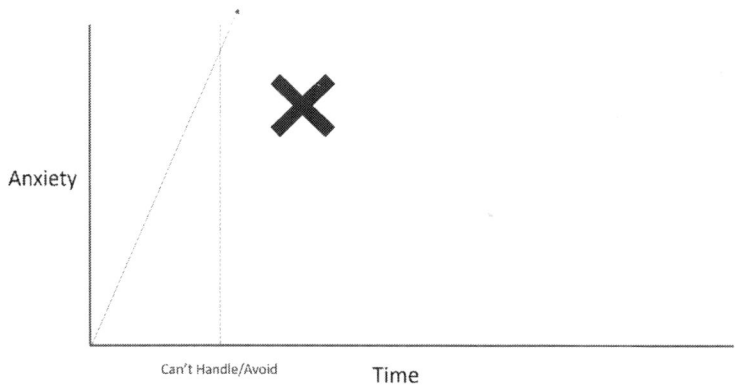

That's why when you leave early, you never really learn that you can handle it. The truth is, you can handle it. You just need time. Anyone who tells me I can't handle [insert social situation], I never believe them. They definitely can, they just don't know it.

You may be wondering then, OK, why would I want to put myself through all that stress and wait a long, long time before I finally feel comfortable and decide to "open up? At first, yes, it seems pretty dumb to put your body through all that anxiety before you start feeling comfortable. But the thing about prolonging your stay in social situations that make you feel uncomfortable is, you teach your subconscious valuable lessons. Your subconscious goes from "Oh no, I'm about to die" mode, to "Oh hey, this ain't so bad" mode. As a result, your peak anxiety levels would, in fact, decrease the next time you face that same situation. In other words, the maximum anxiety level for that social situation would feel less than it was the first time. It would feel more manageable than before. Staying back longer would feel like an easier task. Here's how your anxiety levels would look like over time if you consistently kept facing that same social situation:

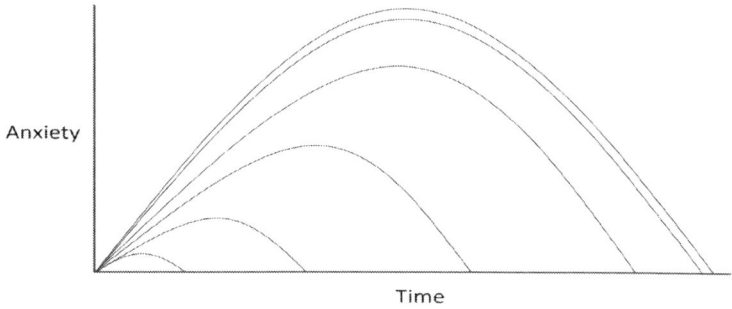

As you can see, when your peak anxiety levels get less and less each time you face the same social situation, you will feel very low anxiety in a shorter amount of time. That is, you would start feeling comfortable and feel less trouble opening up in a shorter amount of time. Also, it wouldn't feel like you are putting your body through deep stress anymore. Eventually, if you keep facing the same social situation many times, you will find that your anxiety levels are really manageable and it will become "just another day" for you.

To reach that level though, you need to be brave and keep exposing yourself to the same social situation you fear very regularly and for a long time. Whether it's going to a party, approaching people, going out for lunch by yourself, speaking over the phone to a stranger, shopping at a mall or whatever. Don't give excuses and say you can't because you need to feed the cat. Go out there, stay long and let your body feel the anxiety as long as it can and then do it again the next day.

When I mentioned "Can't Handle/Avoid" in the graphs, you may be thinking that I mean the said person would be running away from the situation. What I actually mean is avoidance. This includes living and giving some poor excuse for doing so. This also means **safety behaviors**. Things like sitting in the corner of the room hoping not to get noticed, playing on your phone, acting busy, fidgeting with your pockets, sitting awkwardly and so on are also part of avoidance. Any type of avoidance makes your anxiety feel worse the next time. You need to face it head on and just feel the anxiety in full force. It likely WILL feel awkward, uncomfortable, really embarrassing, etc. the first time. But it WILL get better if you keep doing it. Again, go out there, stay long and let your body feel the anxiety as long as it can and then do it again the next day.

I can almost guarantee that this works like a charm. However, saying it is one thing, actually going out there and doing it is another. If you can do this, you are really brave. I mean this from the bottom of my heart. Others may laugh at you when you tell them that you were able to go to a shop and wait in line. Others may think this is no big deal. And they have the right to think like that, since if someone told me they were scared of, I don't know, eggs, I probably wouldn't relate to them. But as someone who has faced social anxiety, I can tell you that you are really brave for attempting to do this. It really isn't easy. There are times where you may feel like giving up. Please don't! Be persistent, at least for the next 3-6 months or so. Treat it as a high priority for now and leave some time every day to practice. If you leave it off for too long, your anxiety levels may come back up again. You need to get it to a very manageable level that even if it comes back up after that, it would take a really long time to do so.

Your social anxiety perhaps took many years to form so it isn't something that's going to cure overnight. Drugs and alcohol can give you temporary relief. But you may feel worse than before once you become sober. It's always better to just be brave and face it head on.

I'd like to make yet another note. While the graphs above seem to show that you will reach 0 anxiety after you stay long enough, this is far from the truth. You will always have a little bit of anxiety. You can't actually get rid of anxiety. This is what your anxiety levels may actually look like:

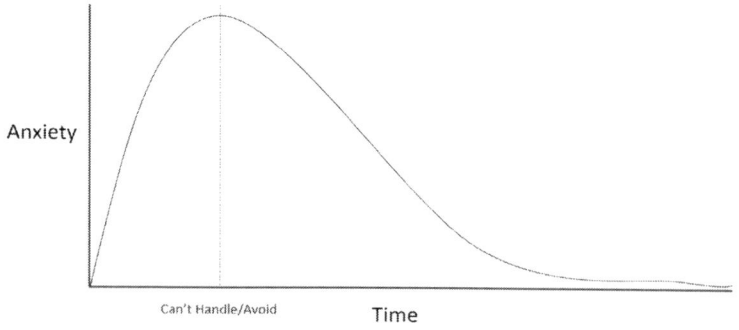

Even though it is not possible to get rid of anxiety, the goal is never to get rid of anxiety. If it were, I would have titled this book "Getting Rid of Social Anxiety and Gaining Confidence". There will always be lingering anxiety but again, this shouldn't stop you from feeling comfortable. The low anxiety level should not get in the way of you opening up. In fact, everyone experiences anxiety when they're out and about. It may be really low to a point that they may not feel it, but it's there. Everyone feels anxious when they meet people for the first time or at a party or whatever. The only difference is, their peak anxiety levels are lower than ours. They can handle it, we can't. Even the most confident of people, such as pop singers, also feel anxiety. I've seen interviews where they say they feel anxiety just before they get up on stage to perform. As they perform many times, they just get comfortable with it even though they're anxious. They may even use that anxiety as fuel to give an electrifying performance. Anxiety can also be beneficial for us in that way.

Breaking The Vicious Cycle

Let's look at our vicious circle diagram again:

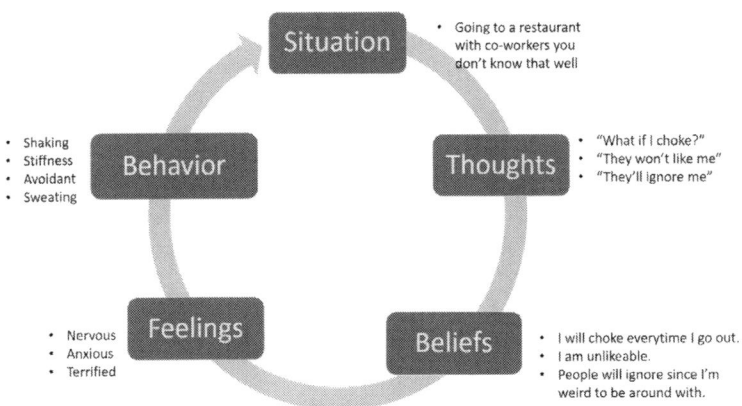

To recap, you're faced with a social situation that you are uncomfortable with. You have constant negative thoughts about the situation. You then develop distorted beliefs about the situation based on your constant negative thoughts as your subconscious has learned and accepted your negative thoughts. You then feel the physical symptoms when you are put in the situation such as heart racing, trembling, etc. This is a vicious cycle that keeps your social anxiety going. It is only when you break this cycle, will you finally start to see improvement.

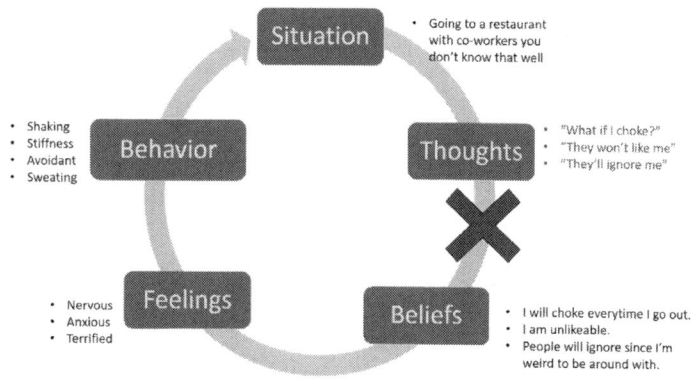

As we mentioned before, this book aims to target your distorted beliefs. Our aim is to not make you think that you're awesome, but to make you **believe** that you're awesome! You have to really believe it. The way we're going to approach this is to change the way we **think**. Out with the negative thoughts, in with the positive. We will deliberately and consciously change the way we think about ourselves in order to change the way we feel about ourselves and in social situations.

How To Change Your Thinking

When we experience social anxiety, we tend to think that we can't cope. We also tend to think that something bad will happen to us. In most cases, this isn't true. In fact, many times, it is quite the opposite. But that is what our subconscious believes. Thus, our negative thinking forces us to think in two different ways:

1. We overestimate the likelihood of something coming true.
2. We underestimate our ability to cope.

These are simply assumptions. We assume something bad will happen to us and we also assume that we won't be able to cope. These assumptions are harmful. It makes us self-conscious and very aware of everything we do. It also changes the way we think about ourselves which in turn affects our self-esteem and self-worth.

Let's look at yet another diagram:

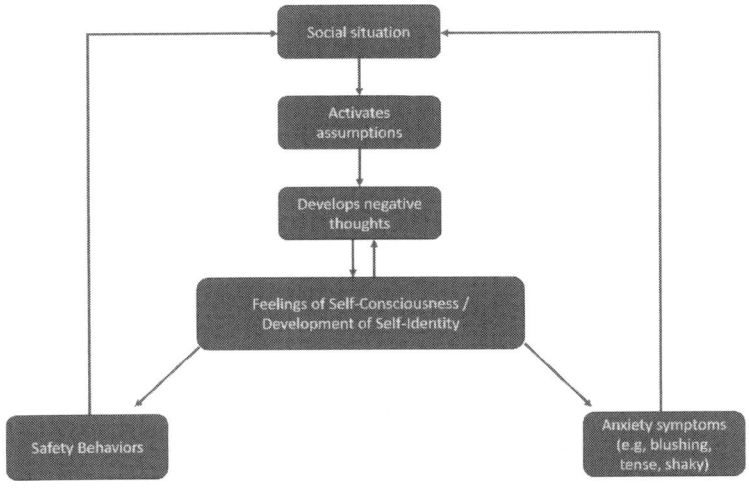

This diagram correlates very much to the vicious cycle. We have a social situation that makes us uncomfortable. That then activates assumptions that the social situation is dangerous and we won't be able to cope and so on. These assumptions make us develop a number of negative thoughts such as "what if I stuff up", "they won't like me", "I'm not worthy of being here" and so on. We then feel really self-conscious of ourselves and the way we behave. We might pay attention to every minute thing that we do (such as moving our arms a little to the left) and feel that people are noticing and judging us badly for it. These negative thoughts affect our beliefs and change the way we see ourselves. This in turn causes us to resort to safety behaviors and/or experiencing anxiety symptoms. This cycle keeps going on and on. The negative thoughts and assumptions become automatic. Your subconscious starts to talk to you. When negative thoughts come to you without you deliberately doing it, it's called *automatic thoughts*. It's in-grained into us. Just like when you watch a movie on repeat 100 times, you may (perhaps subconsciously) keep saying some of the punch dialogues from the film randomly.

To break this cycle, we need to stop assuming. We need to stop assuming bad things will happen to us and we need to understand that we can cope given that we prolong our exposure long enough for the anxiety to go away. Once we stop that, we can then deliberately and consciously challenge our thoughts.

The thing about the subconscious mind is that it can believe things without much evidence. You could actually believe there is a ghost in a dark room without any real evidence other than Hollywood and Japanese movies to support your theory.

When you directly challenge your negative thoughts, your subconscious mind will take notice. When you find yourself in the process of automatic thinking, challenging those negative thoughts will teach your subconscious mind that those thoughts are false. One of the best ways to challenge your negative thoughts is to keep asking yourself "what's the evidence?"

Let's look at some examples below:

- I'm going to stuff up. I might have looked uncomfortable before but there is no actual proof that I stuffed up. That interaction went well. I'm still alive.
- I am unlikeable. She won't talk to me. She hates me. She never once said she hates me. She did mention she was sick though. Maybe that was the reason?
- I don't deserve to be here. I'm less than the others. If I don't deserve to be here, then why was I invited? I must have at least some worth.
- They all think I'm a weirdo. I am odd compared to others. They never called me a weirdo or odd. I'd regard myself as unique. Besides, it's a good thing to be unique.
- I might tip over my drink and everyone will see how clumsy and awkward I am. Fair enough, it is awkward, but this is normal. People spill their

drink all the time. Even if they did see me as clumsy, so what? It's normal.

- They can see me blushing and shaking. They're going to laugh at me/look at me with sympathy. Did they laugh at me? Did they look at me with sympathy? People blush and shake. It's normal. At the end of the day, no-one cares. They would think about more important things rather than care how much I blushed.

See how directly challenging these thoughts can have a positive effect on our thinking and also our beliefs? All of these negative thoughts had no direct evidence that it was true. It's all in our head. When you consistently debunk your negative thoughts, you will notice another shift in subconscious beliefs. Once you develop a strategy to automatically challenge your negative thoughts, your subconscious mind will automatically weed out the rubbish. In addition to improving your anxiety, this will also improve your self-confidence and self-esteem. This is also why I stressed the importance of getting positive and honest feedback from loved ones. They can directly confirm your negative thoughts and prove them wrong. When we are sensitive, the subconscious mind tends to believe others more than our own.

Positive thinking can also help to reverse the effects of negative thinking. Constantly telling yourself that you are awesome, confident, beautiful, and strong and so on can also help. If you can spend a few minutes in front of the mirror every morning complimenting yourself and telling yourself positive things about yourself, you will find that you feel good about yourself and that you love you. Give yourself a smile and a wink before you leave to school or work or wherever.

Low self-esteem can come about from you not liking yourself very much. When you don't love yourself very much, it is too much to expect others to love you. It is only when you love yourself, that you can then expect others to love you. Positive thinking can change that. Continue on Chapter 8 for more information.

In the next chapter, we will be looking at changing our thinking by directly challenging them in a systematic and organized way.

Summary

In this chapter, we looked at the importance of practice and motivation for improving social anxiety as well as getting positive and honest feedback on your progress. We also looked at some truths about our anxiety levels and how they will eventually go down, the longer we stay there. We also looked at how we will approach breaking the vicious cycle. In the next chapter, we will look at finally carrying out the steps in this book systematically and actually exposing ourselves to the situations we fear in an easy and doable way.

Chapter 6

Systematic Way To Overcome Social Anxiety

In this chapter, we will go through and take systematic steps based on CBT which will help us overcome our social anxiety. We first look at generating a stepladder and then working through the stepladder and monitoring your progress. Finally, I'll discuss my own journey in this process.

The Stepladder

It's time to put the cognitive-behavioral techniques discussed in previous chapters into practice and start systematically exposing ourselves to anxiety-provoking social situations. However, we won't be diving into the deep end just yet. The key is to start slow and gradual, allowing ourselves to become comfortable with each step before progressing.

Imagine learning to play the piano. If you only practiced for a day and were then thrust onto a stage to perform a complicated piece in front of thousands, you'd likely become overwhelmed, make mistakes, and perhaps abandon the piano altogether due to that scarring experience. Instead, a gradual approach with incremental steps is far more effective – first performing for an instructor, then family, a larger group, and finally, the big audience. Each step builds confidence and prepares you for the next level.

Similarly, if we were to abruptly expose ourselves to our most feared social situation, like attending a large party, we'd risk feeling awkward, uncomfortable, and potentially discouraged from ever facing that situation again. By gradually working our way up, starting with something relatively simple like walking around a quiet shop with a loved one, we can build our confidence and coping skills step-by-step.

So, let's not rush into anything overwhelming. We'll systematically introduce you to the situations you fear most, but always at your own pace. Overcoming social anxiety takes time, patience, and consistent practice. Trust the process, and don't be discouraged if progress feels slow – every step forward is valuable.

Exercise #1: Identifying Your Fears

To begin, let's create a comprehensive list of all the social situations that cause you anxiety. Open a new spreadsheet and list them out, one by one, as they come to mind. Don't censor yourself – include everything, no matter how minor or severe it may seem. Spend as much time as you need to thoroughly capture all your fears related to social interactions.

Here are some examples to get you started:

- Walking down a public street
- Approaching people
- Eating in front of others
- Talking on the phone with a stranger
- Making small talk
- Telling a joke
- ......

There's no right or wrong answer here really. You might have something completely different. Whatever you fear deep down inside you, just write it down.

If you need more ideas, you can refer to the "My Progress" section of this chapter to see some of the stuff I used to fear.

Exercise #2:

To measure our anxiety level, we will use something called the Subjective Units of Distress Scale (SUDS). This is used by medical professionals to measure the intensity of stress and anxiety that a person feels. The ultimate goal being to measure the effectiveness of treatment for that person over time. Those anxiety graphs I showed you in the previous chapter could be visualized as the SUDS scale of a person over time. To explain simply, SUDS is the level of anxiety ranging from 0 (no anxiety) to 100 (maximum anxiety) you feel about a situation.

Now go ahead and use that list you wrote in Exercise #1, to rank the level of SUDS you feel. You don't need a ruler or some device to measure this. It doesn't have to be exact.

Visualize how anxious you would be in that situation and give yourself a number between 0 (no anxiety) and 100 (most anxiety) about that situation.

Using the example from Exercise #1, here are some SUD ratings:

- Walking down a public street. (20)
- Approaching people. (70)
- Eating in front of people. (75)
- Talking on the phone with a stranger. (60)
- Making small talk. (35)
- Telling a joke. (40)

We can see that eating in front of people and approaching people are the highest since they have a SUD rating of 75 and 70 respectively. These would create a lot of anxiety and best to focus on this last. Walking down a public street has the lowest SUDS rating (20) and thus you will not feel that much anxiety doing this. You would then approach doing this consistently.

Make sure you add the SUDS rating on the second column in Excel. This way, you can use the Excel Sort feature to sort by the second column to see the situation you fear from highest anxiety to lowest anxiety.

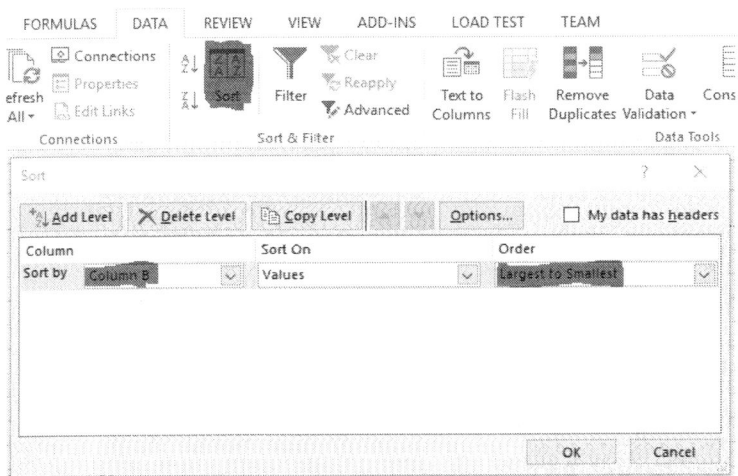

Make sure you also select everything (Ctrl+A) in the spreadsheet before you sort. Make sure you save this file somewhere.

Exercise #3:

If your list is too long, it's time to truncate it. You may have written duplicate entries. Try to group them into something more general. What I mean by that is, say you have entries like "Going to parties", "Going to events", "Going to Comic Con with close friends", could all be grouped simply as "Going to events". Give an average SUDS rating for that. The idea is to shorten the list and make it more general. Something like "Eating alone in public", "Eating with family in public", and "Going out to restaurants with co-workers" could all be grouped as "Eating in public". When you have a shorter list, you can easily work on them one-by-one. I also suggest situations with SUDS rating less than 35 to just get rid of them.

Anxiety levels less than 35 are generally quite manageable. It's not really possible to reduce anxiety to 0. You'll want to focus on the situations that give you noticeable anxiety. It's good to have around 10 items on your list in total but you could have more or less. Do what's comfortable for you.

Again, refer to the "My Progress" section of this chapter to see how I generated my own list of fears.

Gradually Exposing Yourself

It's time to put our plan to action. It's time to expose ourselves to the world! Socially! Look at that final list that you have. Let's start with the situation with the lowest anxiety. Hopefully, it is about 35. In other words, you feel just some level of anxiety. Now go out there and face it, my friend! Face it long, face it hard until that anxiety goes away.

It's normal to feel strong anxiety. In fact, this is completely normal. Stay long enough, and the anxiety WILL start to decrease. Don't run away now. Drop all safety behaviors and don't ever run away. You need to feel the exposure in full force.

If you really can't handle it and the anxiety is too overwhelming, then you need to go back and adjust your SUDS rating. Or better yet, break the current situation into further steps and give them SUDS ratings too.

Let's use our example. The lowest one on that list was making small talk (we ignore walking down a public street since the rating shows it rarely makes us feel anxious). The idea is to now break this down into smaller, more manageable steps.

You could break it down as follows:

- Make small talk. (35)
- Make small talk with strangers with close friends nearby. (30)
- Make small talk with strangers with loved ones nearby. (25)
- Make small talk with other friends with close friends nearby. (20)
- Make small talk with close friends. (15)
- Make small talk with loved ones. (10)

There are many different variations you could try out. Now that you have this broken down, and much more manageable list, you should now practice this every day. That is, every single day, you need to make small talk with the lowest one on the list until you are comfortable. Once you are comfortable, go to the next one on the list and so on and so forth. You will find that once you do this enough times, your anxiety levels will decrease and thus, the SUDS ratings will also decrease. You can take breaks once in a while, but try to do it regularly (at least once a day). If you put it off, you may lose motivation and the anxiety can creep back up again. You'll want to push the SUDS rating to a manageable level and then take a longer break as it would take a longer time for the anxiety to come back.

Monitor Your Thoughts

Once you've exposed yourself to that situation, it's important that you take note of your thoughts. You need to take note of your automatic negative thinking. You would then need to fill out the Thought Monitoring Form. This form is generally used by psychologists and is a part of CBT. This form generally helps you to challenge your negative thinking and rid the distorted beliefs that live in your subconscious. It's important that you fill out this form every single time you carry out the exposure experiment.

You can find many different CBT Thought Monitoring Forms online. The most popular one is from the PsychologyTools website.

Basically, any form that monitors your negative thoughts, anything to challenge those negative thoughts, and give you options to add alternative thoughts. Here is an example:

Situation	Feeling	Negative thought	Evidence	Alternative thought
Approach people	Nervous (60%) Shaking (30%) Blushing (10%)	I will choke	I've choked before. People do choke around new people, it's normal.	They might not care that I choked. They may understand.

Think of your exposure as a social experiment. You want to also observe how others react to you so you could jot this down in the form later to help form your evidence for your negative thoughts. Just like a social experiment, use the opportunity to test the waters and see whether whatever you were fearing about came true or not.

My Negative Thoughts Came True Though

Even if it did come true, so what? Look at the example that I just gave in that Thought Monitoring Form. In the alternative thought column, I wrote "they might not care". If you actually choke, yes, you're fear came true but is it as bad as you think it is? I could have chosen to be positive and write "I might not choke this time" instead, but it's better to be realistic than overly positive all the time.

That's the thing about social anxiety treatment. You will find some of your worst fears coming true. But then you have to keep telling yourself, so what? You have to still keep questioning it. Did you die from the experience? Have people shunned you from society? Most likely not. You could try again the next day and people will most likely not care about it anymore.

The thing about stuffing up and making mistakes, is that it is completely normal. We can't expect to be 100% perfect all the time. We are humans. We make mistakes. It's better to just accept this fact sometimes and just laugh and enjoy these moments rather than catastrophize it as a massive incident. As long as you don't accidentally kill anyone or break any law, you're pretty much good.

Besides, a good fail on your side can sometimes make a good story at the next dinner with friends. You'll have more to talk about!

Helpful Tips

You might find it helps to use ChatGPT for this exercise if you ever feel like you are stuck with your stepladder.

The great thing about Mr ChatGPT, is that he/she is not afraid to challenge your negative thinking.

You can save a lot of time on this exercise by having ChatGPT as your psychologist, but of course, it is by no means a replacement for a real psychologist.

How Long Will It Take Me To Notice A Difference?

The whole process of creating a stepladder, then gradually exposing and rating the anxiety will take time. It's a marathon, not a sprint!

The whole process will help you slowly desensitize you to your source of anxiety.

- **Severity of the Anxiety:** People with severe social anxiety may find it takes longer to progress through the steps of exposure, as each step may require more time to become comfortable with.
- **Consistency and Frequency of Practice:** Regular, consistent exposure exercises can lead to quicker progress. Skipping sessions or not practicing regularly can slow down the process.

- **Support System:** Having a supportive network of friends, family, or a therapist can enhance the effectiveness of the treatment, providing encouragement and motivation. You will have more motivation to stick to things when you have a great and supportive network.
- **Coping Strategies:** Learning and effectively applying coping strategies to manage anxiety can also affect the pace of improvement. Skills like deep breathing, mindfulness, and positive self-talk can make it easier to handle higher SUDS ratings.
- **Individual Differences:** Personal resilience, past experiences, and the presence of other psychological conditions can also impact how quickly someone progresses.

On average, you might start to notice some level of improvement within a few weeks to a few months of doing the exposure tasks.

It's important to approach the process with patience and to set realistic expectations, understanding that progress might also include some setbacks.

It's important to understand that your progress will not be a straight line going upwards. Just like bitcoin, there will be ups and downs. Sometimes you're doing really well and other days, it feel like you've crashed back to 0. But as long as you zoom out and see that you are progressing upwards overall, then you're on the right path.

Personally, I would set a goal for 6 months. Have a stepladder created for each month and stick to it. Honestly, you will be surprised how far you will have reached by the end of the 6th month.

Your anxiety might never go away fully, but you will definitely feel less debilitated than you did at the start!

My Progress

During my social anxiety coping process, I've also followed these steps myself. I will now detail the exact steps I carried out in helping me recover from social anxiety.

The Stepladder

First, I listed all the social situations that made me afraid in an Excel spreadsheet and gave them a SUDS rating between 0 and 100 where 0 indicated the lowest fear and 100 indicated the highest fear. Here is the list below:

- Giving a compliment to someone (54)
- Looking away when speaking (38)
- Showing an interest in others' lives (63)
- Asking for directions (42)
- Eating in public (80)
- Meeting new people (50)
- Having a conversation with others (80)
- Sitting in a park by myself (10)
- Being complimented (5)
- Speaking on the phone with a stranger (67)
- Saying hello/goodbye to people at work (66)

- Being watched when doing nothing (85)
- Going to a crowded shopping mall (70)
- Being assertive, saying "no" (90)
- Going to parties (75)
- Giving a speech (95)
- Job interviews (81)
- Group meetings (92)
- Going to restaurant with co-workers (88)

After this, I used Excel's Sort feature to sort the list based on my SUDS rating. I ordered it from highest anxiety to lowest anxiety.

- Giving a speech (95)
- Group meetings (92)
- Being assertive and saying "No" (90)
- Going to the restaurant with co-workers (88)
- Being watched when doing nothing (85)
- Job interviews (81)
- Eating in public (80)
- Having a conversation with others (80)
- Going to parties (75)
- Going to a crowded shopping mall (70)
- Saying hello/goodbye to people at work (66)
- Showing an interest in others' lives (63)
- Giving a compliment to someone (54)
- Meeting new people (50)
- Asking for directions (42)
- Looking away when speaking (38)

- Sitting in a park by myself (10)
- Being complimented (5)

I then decided which ones I wanted to work on for the next couple of months. I ruled out the first few ones such as being complimented or sitting in a park by myself since my anxiety was low enough already and I couldn't possibly get 0 anxiety. I was comfortable enough with it. I narrowed it to the most important ones that I wanted to work on as below:

- Giving a speech (95)
- Group meetings (92)
- Being assertive (90)
- Eating in public (85)
- Having a conversation with others (80)
- Going to parties (75)
- Going to a crowded shopping mall (70)
- Speaking on the phone with a stranger (67)
- Saying hello/goodbye to people at work (66)

Now, I started from the lowest; Saying hello/goodbye to people at work. This was something I was a bit nervous about. I couldn't just go up the next day and just say hello or goodbye to them. It made me really nervous. I usually nod or mumble whenever they say hi/bye to me, but I never initiated it myself. So, what did I do? I broke this step into further steps as follows:

- Say hello/goodbye to people at work (66)
- Say hello/goodbye to people at work that I'm most comfortable with (55)

- Say hello/goodbye to relatives (50)
- Say hello/goodbye to relatives in front of family (40)
- Say hello/goodbye to friends (30)
- Say hello/goodbye to family (20)

Easy enough. I then chipped away working on this task for a couple of weeks. I would consistently say hi/bye to my family and after a week, I got used to it. I then slowly tried the same thing with my friends. It was awkward at first, but I got used to it. Eventually, I made my way to the top. It was actually awkward. There were times where people didn't respond back. This is where negative thoughts came into play and I was able to catch a few of them.

- They didn't say hi back. They hate me.
- They think I'm weird.
- I am unlikeable.
- Don't say hi. They didn't respond last time.
- I must have offended them somehow.
- Why does this only happen to me?

Wow, no wonder I had so much anxiety and distorted beliefs. I then debunked those thoughts using the Thought Monitoring Form as follows:

Situation	Feeling	Negative thought	Evidence	Alternative thought
Say hi/bye to people at work	Nervous (60%) Shaking (30%) Blushing (10%)	They hate me.	They never said they hate me.	They like me. They could be neutral.
		They think I'm weird.	I don't know if they think I'm weird. They did look at me funny though.	They may be impressed that I said "hi".
		I am unlikeable.	They never said that. They never told me to go away.	I am likable.
		I must have offended them	They didn't respond last time.	They were probably busy.
		Why does this only happen to me?	It happens to others too. This is a wrong statement.	This happens to a lot of people. This is normal. No big deal.

I then kept doing this every day until I got comfortable with it. In other words, until that SUDS rating dropped below 30. Remember, it is not possible to reach an anxiety level of 0. It was important that I filled out the Thought Monitoring Form daily. I couldn't let my negative thoughts get the upper hand on me. I needed to debunk it as soon as I got home.

Once I felt comfortable with this, I then moved onto the next thing on my stepladder; speaking on the phone with a stranger.

It has worked well for me thus far. I'm really thankful for having a good support system along the way. My close family have been instrumental in giving me positive and honest feedback which has only helped me get better. Some of the members from the social club I attend (will explain in the next chapter) have also helped decrease my anxiety and increase my confidence in social situations.

At the time of writing, I am at a point where I'm trying to nail Giving a Speech and Group Meetings. These ones are a lot more challenging because you just don't do them every day. It's not like you can go crash into some lecture hall and hope people will listen to you. Some ways I'm approaching this for the speech one, is giving video tutorials on YouTube regarding animation (a topic I'm really interested in). That, however, isn't the same as giving a speech in front of a live audience.

Summary

In this chapter, we learnt about the stepladder and gradual exposure. We listed out the social situations that make us uncomfortable. We then ranked the situations based on SUDS and systematically looked at challenging our negative thinking but questioning our negative thoughts on a Thought Monitoring Form. I also briefly explained my own process. In the next chapter, we will look at ways to gain self-confidence and feel awesome about yourself!

Chapter 7

Improving Self-Confidence

In this chapter, we will look at ways to improve our self-confidence. While we have been focusing thus far on drastically reducing our social anxiety, we may still have low self-esteem and low self-confidence. We will discuss how focusing on social skills as well as doing the things we love helps improve our self-confidence. We also look at utilizing social anxiety groups and Toast-masters for further social exposure as well as gaining self-confidence.

Develop Social Skills

When we don't have much social interaction with others, we become out of touch with social skills. We start to lose our ability to make small talk or know how to keep a conversation going. All the other stuff I taught you in the other chapters are great at helping you get rid of your social anxiety. However, it doesn't help you suddenly become sociable. In other words, while you may start to feel comfortable approaching people, you may not know what to say or how to keep the other person engaged.

It's no good approaching a random person with confidence to say "Hi" and then stay dead silent for the next 3 hours while facing him. That would make it awkward for you and most likely for him too.

Once you start to get a little comfortable with social situations, you should take some time to develop social skills. In other words, skills that help us to communicate effectively with other people through our words, body language and gestures. Having good social skills makes it easy for people to approach you and get comfortable around you. The other benefit of good social skills is that it can definitely help improve your self-confidence. The better you get at socializing with others, the better you get at developing your style and personality. This helps you develop your own self-image and makes you confident. Let's now look at some ways you can develop good social skills:

Reading About It

There are countless tutorials on the web teaching you how to develop good social skills. They cover everything imaginable, from body language to conversing effectively to jokes, small talk and so on. It would help if you could find time to do some reading into some of this stuff. Then study it and try it out in the real world. Use the SUDS scale if you have to. There is not enough scope in this book to teach you all this stuff since it requires its own books.

Due to your social anxiety, you may not have had much social interaction with people and thus, you may have lost touch. Reading about this stuff can give you more insight and help you re-learn the skills you may have lost after your social anxiety takeover.

Socialize More

Take as much opportunity as possible to keep socializing with others. Just like with the gradual and long exposure method, try to force yourself to have conversations with people every day. That's right, every day. Even better if you can have a long conversation every day. A time waste? Probably. But it needs to be done. The longer you converse every day, the more your anxiety will improve and on top of that, the more you will learn *how* to converse effectively. It doesn't matter who you socialize with; your close friends, your close family, your dog, your imaginary friend (if you still have one) or even that character from your favorite computer game. I don't really recommend the latter though.

Start off slow and at a pace that you're comfortable with. Use the SUDS scale if you can't handle it initially. Start with speaking with your close family/friends, then slowly make your way up to strangers. Remember, you've only just decided to fight your social anxiety. So, initial "fails" and "awkward" moments are kind of inevitable. This is OK. The more you do it, the less you will experience those moments. And once you start getting comfortable with socializing, you may even start to laugh at your own failures and awkward moments. Laughing at your own mistakes can make you much more likable to others as they see you as a person who is real and human. Laughing at your own mistakes also makes you more resilient to failure, and shows that you have an upper hand over your own distorted beliefs.

You should use any socializing opportunity to observe and see how people react to you. No, I don't mean that whole "What are they gonna think of me? They hate me" kind of observation. I mean, just casually observe. If you genuinely sense someone is in a hurry, or they want to end the conversation, then end it smoothly without wasting much of their time. If you see that they are really interested in your story, then keep it going instead of cutting it short to one sentence only. Learning to pick up little cues like that from people makes you a lot more approachable by other people usually. By socializing regularly, you will automatically learn to pick up all these cues and see what parts of your current social skills work well and what doesn't. You can then improve on those. Sometimes you may make mistakes. Then again, as long as you continue socializing, you will automatically learn to accept those mistakes and move on.

A lot of people don't realize this, but socializing is also a skill. Just like playing the piano, or playing a game of cricket. You can't just go in and expect to nail it on the first go. You need practice. And the more practice you get, the better you will get. You need to try it out for yourself to believe.

Just Listen

Listening is a very valuable skill. What you may not realize, is that listening can be such a powerful tool. People may not care or become curious that you are too quiet if they see that you are listening to them.

Another good thing about listening, is that it gives you the ample opportunity to learn how others socialize. When you are in a group with people who socialize well, it can be helpful once in a while, to not put so much pressure on yourself and just observe how others do it. Listening in on another group's conversation while you are pretending to do some work on your own can help you see how others approach conversation and make jokes and whatever. I don't condone this that much however, as it can be a little weird and stalker-ish doing so.

Try to observe someone whose socializing abilities you admire. You might admire their friendliness, their approachability and the ease with how they make you feel comfortable to open up around them. Try to break down and analyze how they do it and then try to emulate it. Don't ever try to become that person, since that will lose your own self-identity. Instead, grab some of their skills and make it your own. I'm sure there's no copyright law thingy for that.

Keep Up-To-Date With News

This might seem like mundane homework. Try to keep yourself up-to-date with the latest news, movies, weather and so on.

When you keep yourself up-to-date with the latest, you not only appear knowledgeable and aware, but you now have more topics to discuss when you socialize with people.

I don't suggest keeping up-to-date with news as if it was homework. Just do what feels natural to you. If you're interested in that news, dig deeper and find some cool facts. If you don't care, don't force yourself to care.

Doing Things You Love

While focusing on improving your social skills is definitely a good thing, it doesn't help to always focus on socializing and finding ways to improve your social anxiety. Every once in a while, you need to get away from all that and think about yourself. Do whatever it is that you enjoy. Whether it's watching a movie, reading a good book, or going to a park, make sure it's also a part of your daily schedule. Just like it's unhealthy to always work, work, work and no fun. You need to find that balance. And doing the things you love can balance things out. You need that release.

The thing that helps me is spending quality time with close family and friends, watching YouTube videos and spending Saturday mornings at a quiet park. Those things give me a release from a stressful day. When you practice gradual exposure, you will feel a lot of stress. Equally, you need something to release that stress. Unfortunately, I can't help you in finding what releases you. Only you would know that. Whatever makes you feel calm and sort of happy is pretty much the release that you're looking for. You'll need to make sure to do that regularly as well. A calmer mind might not give you self-confidence, but it makes the journey of getting there a more pleasant one.

If you want to develop self-confidence out of doing the things you love, you need to find something you feel you are really good at. Whether it's a hobby like fishing or sport, make sure you spend time developing those extra skills. Achieving those skills and becoming really good at it, can generally make you self-confident. Personally, I make movies for YouTube. Only recently have I started getting really good at it and it's always nice to see the positive comments for my work. I was also selected for a screening for a short film festival for one of my short films. Making movies has generally raised my self-confidence to much more than what I expected. It has made me feel like I'm worth much more than what I initially thought.

Others have gained self-confidence through working out and getting a nicely shaped body. I personally met someone from Toastmasters who used to be really shy and uncon- fident. After working out and getting a better physique, he changed. All that energy and endorphins have done won- ders to his self-confidence.

Other ideas could include teaching, playing a musical instrument, singing, sports, gaming to name a few. Try to develop your talent in any of these and stop thinking about social anxiety all the time. Developing these skills is also similar to those graphs of social anxiety. Initially, in those learning periods, you don't feel much progress. Once you hit that threshold, you start to accelerate and learn things at a rapid pace. Doing the things you love and developing those skills can do great wonders to your self-confidence. Believe me when I say this. On top of that, it also generally makes you feel good. Even if you aren't progressing that much in your social anxiety journey, you still feel that life is good and that there is something to look forward to the next day. If you do become awesome at something, flaunt it without shame but don't let it get too much to your head!

Joining Clubs

Try to find some clubs where you enjoy what they do and what they have to do. If you like painting, join a painting club. If you like comics, join a comic club. The good thing about these clubs is that you get to find a lot of like-minded people and getting friends (and possibly a mate) would be a lot easier. You don't need to worry about being stuck yet again in a group where you don't fit in.

Attending Social Anxiety Groups

In order to tackle social anxiety and then gain self-confidence, you need repeated exposure to social situations. That's not all. You need to socialize with people till you're comfortable. If you were like me, and struggled to start socializing, it may be because you're putting yourself in a social situation in which you aren't ready yet. Using the stepladder, you can start small. You could socialize with your close family members and then make your way up.

If you'd like to start out easy, you could try your local social anxiety support group. Generally, if you live in a country where social anxiety issues are quite common (which are mostly western countries), you would likely find a social anxiety support group near where you live. Just Google

"Social Anxiety Support Group [Insert where you live]" and you may find some.

These are generally small, focused groups who meet on a regular schedule for 1 or 2 hours and discuss ways to tackle social anxiety. These groups also generally tend to be free. This is a great place to start your stepladder. You get to meet people who also have the same social anxiety issues you have. This can also make you feel better about yourself, knowing that you're not the only one out there. There are others who are just as awkward and/or uncomfortable with social situations as you are. This can be quite confidence boosting.

Social Anxiety Support groups are a great place to start your stepladder journey, since you get the exposure to social situations with relatable people in an easy and warm environment. It should be a warm environment. After all, it is a support group full of sensitive people like us. You're also forced to speak by the psychologist in charge of the sessions, so you don't need to wait for the right moment to contribute or anything like that. It should generally be easy. Initially though, it is quite nerve-wracking to enter that room, but once you meet some of the people there, you may actually look forward to the experience.

I'd recommend going for around 8 sessions or so. This gives you plenty of exposure with strangers and the chance to persistently socialize with them. Who knows, by the end of these sessions, you may be a lot more confident than you initially imagined.

Toastmasters

This is another great place to get regular social exposure and gain self-confidence. Toastmasters is a non-profit organization focused on communication and leadership development. Their aim is to help members become confident public speakers in a warm, friendly and supportive environment. Basically, it's a club you can join to practice public speaking skills regularly. The idea is to make you feel comfortable with public speaking by actually making you speak in front of an audience.

There are usually weekly (or fortnightly) meetings where members get together and present speeches on whatever they want. They then evaluate speeches and give them constructive feedback for improvement. Toastmaster clubs are located everywhere in the world. It's seriously popular but still, not a lot of people know about it. You can go onto the Toastmasters website and see where the nearest club is to you. You may be surprised how close you are to one. There are literally thousands of clubs around the world. If not, you can always start your own.

I remember when my psychologist strongly recommended that I joined. I was barely 5 sessions in, and he pushed me to join. A bit of a massive leap. Here I was, still fearing going to the nearest post office myself, and pretty much told I'm ready to handle public speaking and that I should start with that on my stepladder. I still remember that first day. It was weird because my psychologist pumped me up and made me excited to go, but on the actual day I kept thinking about it. What if I look weird? I'm going to be so out of place. I don't know if I even deserve to be here. I had a range of crazy thoughts like that. I remember I parked my car and walked to the entrance of the building. The door was locked. I tried to open it, still locked. I felt a little relieved and even contemplated going home and telling myself "At least I tried". I knew that was a poor excuse, so I went around the building and found the entrance was there instead. My nerves creeped up and I just went in. I was greeted by a number of enthusiastic members who cheered as soon as I walked in (they knew I was coming since I emailed two days earlier). They made me feel comfortable and even convinced me to join. Till now, I feel that Toastmasters was one of the richest experiences I felt in my life changing social journey.

A meeting would generally run for 2 - 3 hours depending on which club you attend. Each club is so different from another. My one went for 3 hours. The first hour would be Table Topics. These are pretty much impromptu speeches. This is the most nerve-wracking one for all members. One member comes up and brings up a random topic and assigns another random member to talk about it for 1 - 2 minutes without any preparation. It can also be fun since there is no pressure to get it right. You can make up the weirdest stuff, since all they judge you on is your confidence and the way you deliver your speech. Then, the next 15 minutes or so, would be a short break with refreshments. I had many opportunities here to meet with other members and get to know them. This was also a great time to practice small talk. People do approach you and are quite friendly. It was really interesting now that I think about it. I met people who had vastly different dreams and outlook on life. They even made me comfortable to open up and share a bit of my own life. The remaining hours would be spent on the Prepared Speeches. This is where members would present a speech they have been preparing since the last meeting. One of the members in the club is assigned as your mentor and will help you prepare for and deliver your speech. I had 2 mentors and both were really friendly. They would invite me over to their house every week to help me rehearse my speech and give me constructive feedback. This would set me up for the Prepared Speeches part of the Toastmasters meeting.

The Prepared Speeches usually go for 5 – 7 minutes and a great time to get that social exposure. 5 – 7 minutes is quite a long time when you're standing out in front and everyone is staring at you. I noticed my anxiety would be really high at the start of the speech but would die down halfway when I see people being receptive to it. This prolonged exposure helped me notice my anxiety getting less, the longer I spoke. At the end of the meetings, members would evaluate your speech (both the impromptu ones and the prepared ones). They would also give you constructive feedback. It is through the feedback, did I find encouragement. I learnt that I appeared confident from the outside even though I was freaking out inside. I was told I was a little quiet though but it is something that I could improve. This, I believe, gave me a lot of self-confidence. With each meeting, the positive feedback and reinforcement helped slowly change my subconscious thinking about the way I think about myself and others.

I personally think Toastmasters is a great place to start your stepladder journey. It's easy, people are generally alright with your nervousness and won't call you out or make you feel uncomfortable for it, they're all really friendly and supportive (at least my one was), and you get your own personal mentor who can become your best friend and can be a part of your journey to self-confidence. I really think Toastmasters is a great place to start tackling social anxiety, even if you think you aren't ready. I think I sound a little sales-y. I promise I don't work for or get any commissions from Toastmasters or anything like that.

Membership does cost you and it's around $120 per year or so which isn't that expensive compared to seeing a psychologist or something. You get loads of material regarding how to prepare your speeches, body language as well as how to gain confidence when speaking. The stuff I mentioned earlier about you needing to learn social skills by reading stuff. You get a lot of that reading material by joining and on top of that, you get to practice what you've read in an easy-going social environment. I started to gain confidence around my 20th speech. Just a reference for those who don't see much returns after their second meeting or so. It's alright to fail. Saying the wrong thing or choking will not scar you a lot in this environment. In fact, it is normal to see others who also look uncomfortable and choke on their words as well. It's just love and compassion for one another.

Seeing a Psychologist

If you still find all this quite challenging, your next best option would be to go see a psychologist. A psychologist can work with you to identify the real cause of your social anxiety and may help you form a stepladder which is more targeted to you.

I had also seen a psychologist myself. In fact, I don't think I would have followed through with my step ladder without the help of a psychologist. They can really motivate you and push you to continue when your energy levels are down socially.

The best thing about seeing a psychologist is that this is another opportunity to get more social exposure. You can practice socializing with your own psychologist. Generally, psychologists would work with you and do things like role-playing to help you visualize yourself in that social situation and give you a sort of dress-rehearsal for the real thing. If you see your psychologists very regularly (say weekly), you can gain a lot out of it. Just make sure you have enough cash in the bank because they do charge for each session.

Again, if your social anxiety issues are a lot worse than that, in the sense that it is deeply impacting your life, it would be best to see a psychiatrist instead. This book may not help that much. Psychiatrists can prescribe medication which can help you temporarily cope. I advise that you see a psychologist first and see what they think before deciding to see a psychiatrist. Medication for social anxiety has side effects and it's best to avoid it, unless you really need it.

Summary

In this chapter, we looked at ways to improve our self-confidence and self-esteem. We looked at focusing on developing social skills as well as other unrelated skills that we have a passion for. We also looked at utilizing social anxiety support groups, Toastmasters and a personal psychologist to help you drastically reduce social anxiety and gain self-confidence.

Chapter 8

Conclusion

In this chapter, we review everything we've learned from this book and conclude the book.

So What Did We Learn?

Let's go chapter-by-chapter and review what we've learned.

- In Chapter 1, we looked at what social anxiety is and how it is caused. I also gave a bit of a background with how social anxiety came about for me.
- In Chapter 2, we learnt about how thoughts, feelings and actions are linked and how constantly thinking negatively can affect our subconscious thinking which causes us to feel fear in social situations.
- In Chapter 3, we learnt about what kept our social anxiety going. We particularly learnt that avoidance was the main culprit, and that any form of avoidance, whether it was direct or indirect via safety behaviors, makes our social anxiety worse.

- In Chapter 4, we looked at ways to cope with social anxiety symptoms such as deliberately slowing your breathing, shifting attention away and spending time doing things that relax you.
- In Chapter 5, we looked at what will reduce our social anxiety overall. We stressed the importance of practice and to do it consistently to get great results as well as the importance of positive and honest feedback. We also looked at some truths about our coping ability and our improvement over time. We learnt that our anxiety will gradually get less, the more we face that social situation for a prolonged period when we're there. We also learnt that positive self-dialogue when we notice ourselves negatively thinking can change our distorted subconscious thinking.
- In Chapter 6, we looked at how to systematically start tackling our social anxiety. We were introduced to the stepladder and how to go about gradually exposing ourselves to the things we fear. If our stepladder was still too much, we knew we could break it down further. We also learnt that we needed to face this situation regularly until our anxiety reaches a manageable level.
- In Chapter 7, we looked at ways to gain self-confidence. I suggested going to social anxiety support groups, participating in Toastmaster meetings, and seeing a psychologist. I also suggested developing your social skills through

socializing more and reading good books and guides about it.

Last Bits of Advice

Hopefully by now, you will have a better understanding of how you can go about tackling social anxiety. But don't just sit there and expect good things to happen. Go out there and face your fear. Your real journey begins now. It will be a tough journey. You will face so much failure in terms of embarrassment, rejection, awkwardness and at the same time you will face so much success in terms of realizing how confident and brave you really are, which may result in newer friendships and opportunities in your life. The success will almost certainly outweigh the failures on your journey. And that too by a big margin.

This book may have been a stepping stone for you to get started. From here on in, it is up to you to execute this into action. You have the skills now. You also have the tools now. And you also have the knowledge now. Continue to build upon these and keep learning, practicing and experimenting. Don't ever worry about failing. It's all part of the process of learning and growing. Remember, it's like learning to ride your bike or playing a piano. Don't go all out. Just take it one step at a time at your own pace.

The first few months are going to be tough. You need to be brave during this time. You need to be really courageous and fight this through. Eventually, you will hit that threshold or that "A-ha!" moment, and from thereon, it gets easier and easier. Still, you can't stop. Go to the next stage of your stepladder and try to tackle that. Remember to also leave aside some time each day to do the things that you love and the things that relax you, whether that's watching a movie or sitting at a nice park on a Saturday morning. Rewarding yourself is a good way to show that you love yourself.

Even though social anxiety has been around for a while, research in how to tackle it has been quite new. Research is active in this area as social anxiety becomes more prevalent in a society where people are always on their phones and social connections are mostly made online. With the growing popularity of virtual reality, social anxiety will be on the rise and social skills will start to decline. I do expect there will be more groundbreaking research and breakthroughs in how to tackle this problem but we'll never know for sure how the next ten years pan out. You have a great opportunity now more than ever to improve your social anxiety and gain self-confidence. In a world where digitization seems to rule, there is also a growth in the number of social clubs, and socializing events which you can make full use of to practice your social skills, reduce your social anxiety and ultimately make more connections with real people and get opportunities, ideas and perspectives that you would never have thought about.

You're never too early or too late to start. The best time to start is now.

If you want to continue learning with me, I encourage you to connect with me at CalmKavi.com by subscribing to my email list. Whenever I learn something useful, I will be happy to share it with you for free! There's also a ton of posts right now which may be useful to your learning process.

That's It!

Well done! Now you've officially reached the end of the book. It has been my pleasure to teach and share with you the skills needed to tackle social anxiety. I had structured this book in a way that would be beneficial to helping you learn and maximize your potential to improve your social anxiety and gaining self-confidence. I hope you had a lot of fun reading and following this book and that it at least helped you out a little bit in your journey.

Let's keep in contact as I will bring you more helpful and affordable books in future. If you subscribe to my email list, you will get future books for free.

Just before I sign off, I just wanted to, again, say congratulations! You've just passed the first stage of your social anxiety conquering journey. You're now set and well on your way to true self-confidence!

Thank you for reading, and good luck! ☺

About the Author

Danio Kavi is a software engineer/writer/filmmaker/educator. His goal is to help as many people as possible who suffer from social anxiety and social phobia related issues. Danio had also suffered from social anxiety issues preventing him from progressing in life and is now on a path to gain self-confidence. He hopes to one day inspire other people to bring out the best version of themselves and help them achieve success in their life.

One Last Thing...

If you enjoyed this book or found it useful I'd be very grateful if you'd post a short review on Amazon. Your support really does make a difference and I read all the reviews personally so I can get your feedback and make this book even better.

Thanks again for your support!

Made in the USA
Columbia, SC
30 December 2024

50887844R00072